.a doctor discusses

learning to cope with arthritis, rheumatism and gout

By Robert E. Dunbar, M.S.J.

Fellow, American Medical Writers Association

In Consultation with

HAROLD F. SEEGALL, M.D.

BUDLONG PRESS COMPANY • 5428 N. Virginia Avenue • Chicago, Illinois 60625

Acknowledgement To The Consultant

The author is indebted to Dr. Harold F. Seegall who, in his role as consultant, devoted a great deal of time and thought to this manuscript. Dr. Seegall suggested many revisions to make this book as comprehensive and helpful as possible to the arthritic patient.

In his 36 years of practice Dr. Seegall has had considerable success in treating arthritic patients who have permitted themselves the benefit of proper management of their disease. He is a firm believer in patient management, particularly in the case of chronic illnesses such as arthritis. Treatment can not be casual; it must be regular and over a long period of time.

Dr. Seegall also believes that the mental attitude of the patient is of primary importance. No matter how severe or painful his arthritic condition may be, the patient should adopt an optimistic attitude for his own benefit. He can be helped. With proper management the arthritic patient can enjoy a useful, productive, and relatively happy life.

ILLUSTRATIONS BY DAN W. LOTTS

Table of Contents

A Disease As Old As Man

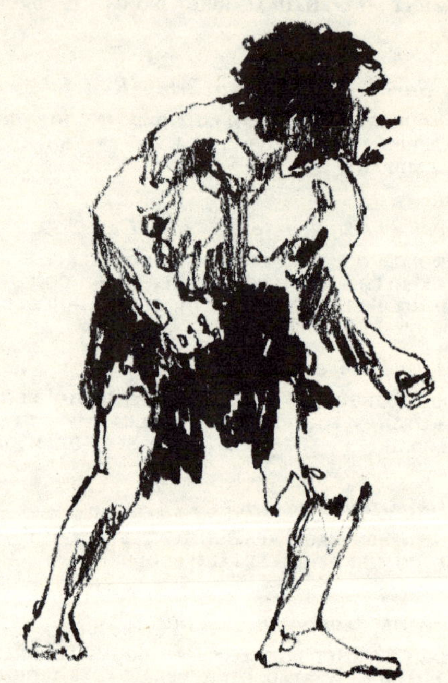

Arthritis, rheumatoid arthritis and gout all belong in the same family of chronic rheumatic diseases. They share similarities, and they have important and marked differences. One thing they all have in common is that they have plagued man from the beginning of time.

The famous philosopher, Socrates of ancient Greece, placed arthritis first among the common diseases of his era. During the days of the Roman Empire the disease was so prevalent that the Emperor Diocletian had an edict proclaimed that exempted those who were seriously afflicted from payment of taxes!

Many of the most famous men and women of history have suffered the vicissitudes and discomforts of arthritis, rheumatoid arthritis or gout, among them: Julius Caesar, Louis XIV, Frederick the Great, John Calvin, William Pitt, Catherine de Medici, Mary Queen of Scots, and probably one of the best known, through literature, movies, and television, Henry the 8th of England.

These are chronic illnesses that are still very much with us, to which tens of millions throughout the world can testify.

The author hopes this book will help you and your family to better understand your illness and how you can learn to cope with it successfully under your physician's direction.

There are many ways in which you can be helped. There is medication which your physician will prescribe, depending on the state your condition is in. There are exercises, recommended rest periods, self-help devices to make you feel more comfortable. And if your condition warrants it, your physician may recommend surgery to correct a painful condition that cannot be helped in any other way.

The important thing to keep in mind is to faithfully follow your physician's advice. Don't, under any circumstances, be misled or duped by extravagant claims from any source that promise you a "miraculous" cure and sudden end to your condition. There is no known cure at this writing for arthritis, rheumatoid arthritis or gout. But you can be helped— very significantly—and that's what this book is all about.

CHAPTER 1

Millions of Fellow Sufferers

Of one thing you can be certain: you are not alone in your discomfort and pain with arthritis. According to the National Health Education Committee, Inc., at least 10 million Americans suffer from osteoarthritis, five million from rheumatoid arthritis, and one million from gout. The Canadian figures are no more encouraging. There are probably many millions more with a mild or untreated form of one of these chronic illnesses.

The Arthritis Foundation has stated that "Almost everyone, if he lives long enough, will develop some arthritis. Studies show that 97 per cent of all individuals over age 60 have enough arthritis so that it can be seen in x-ray films."

Arthritis, rheumatism, and gout are not diseases of the old. These diseases can strike at any age, even in infancy and often in the prime of life. If left untreated, they can become progressively worse, eventually leading to painful crippling. This is particularly true in the case of rheumatoid arthritis, which can destroy the joints unless effective treatment is administered in time.

Because arthritis is so common there is a tendency among non-sufferers—even those who have minor complaints—to treat the illness lightly. This is a serious mistake. In its early stages, arthritis may start with only minor aches and pains. But left untreated or ignored it can lead to serious illness, extreme pain, and even to permanent deformities of the hands, wrists, knees, feet or hips. Without proper treatment arthritis can become so severe that the sufferer must be bedridden for life or dependent on a wheelchair. Think what this would mean to a family, emotionally and economically. And in the great majority of cases it is unnecessary.

People who believe that nothing much can be done for arthritis are only fooling themselves. A great deal can be done, and the future holds promise that even more can be done for those who start treatment early and continue to follow their doctor's advice. Crippling is not inevitable, even in the most serious cases. And if it does occur it can be reduced and corrected.

Must arthritis victims suffer pain? Yes, some pain cannot be avoided. But it can be controlled and alleviated. Again, the necessity for early and regular treatment by a qualified physician can't be emphasized strongly enough. If the victim or sufferer acts in time he can prevent irreversible damage to his joints.

Don't listen to bad advice from people who are misinformed about arthritis. Have you ever heard comments like, "It's just rheumatism. The pain will probably go away in a couple of days. Why should you go to the doctor? He'll only tell you to take some aspirin. They can't do much for arthritis anyway."

Don't pay any attention to these comments. And avoid home remedies like the plague. Take your complaints to your doctor—without delay.

Arthritis is a serious disease. The earlier you begin treatment the better the chances are that you will avoid pain, disability, and lifelong handicaps. The Arthritis Foundation puts it this way:

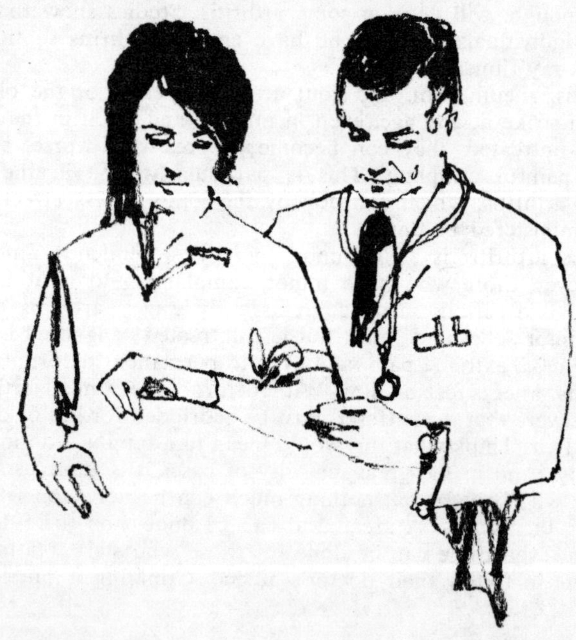

"When medical emergencies strike, we rush to our doctors and trust them to perform overnight miracles. The problem is acute . . . and medicine is geared to go into action quickly. We expect the crisis to be over in a matter of hours.

"Chronic disease—and arthritis is the most widespread example—is something else. Once you have arthritis, chances are you're stuck with it for life. You might as well learn to adjust to it, for better or worse, just the way you accept the shape of your nose or your height or anything else you were born with that you don't particularly like.

"Chronic arthritis comes on slowly, gets worse slowly and, even with the best of treatment, gets better slowly. Don't look for quick, dramatic answers to it, because there are none."

Once you begin treatment and management under a physician's supervision you *can* expect improvement—not quickly and dramatically, in most cases, but over a period of time, depending on the extent of your condition. This is something you must have faith in. Don't be discouraged by the fact that there is no instant cure or quick end to pain and discomfort. Have patience, and follow your doctor's advice. Improvement will come in time, and much of the improvement that will come will depend on *you*.

The better you understand your condition, the more you will be able to adjust to it. It will also help if your family understands your illness.

The person who suffers from arthritis or any rheumatic disease is well aware of the unstableness of his condition. In the morning the pain and stiffness can be almost unbearable. But after a few hours the pain and stiffness lessen and you begin to feel better. By evening, however, the pain and stiffness return.

You can even enjoy long periods of a week or more when you aren't bothered at all by your arthritis. Then it suddenly returns with a vengeance. It's a strange disease in that you are not always aware of its presence. But it is always there.

This can affect you emotionally. You enjoy the periods when you're not aware of the pain and stiffness. But when they suddenly strike again, you may become depressed and irritable. Your family doesn't have to treat you like an invalid, and you don't want them to feel that you are. But a little understanding can help you feel better.

One way to maintain good spirits is to keep involved in family affairs and to keep doing interesting things, in spite of any discomfort you may feel. The worse thing you can do is to give in to self-pity. This will only make you feel worse.

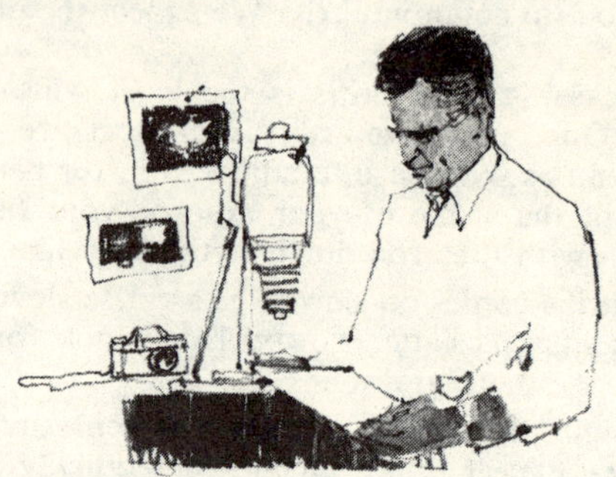

Hobbies are recommended as a means of helping to take your mind off the discomforts of arthritis.

Arthritis management is usually two-phased. Like a burning fire, it must first be put out and care taken that there are no glowing embers left behind which might rekindle an active fire. Once the fire is put out then the rebuilding (rehabilitation) can begin.

At times putting out the fire can be a fairly rapid process; while at other times, because of a tendency to rekindling, it may be quite some time before it is confined. It is unfortunate that by the time many people with arthritis see a doctor their arthritic condition has reached the stage where rehabilitation is of great importance. This rebuilding process can be quite slow. Destroyed materials may first have to be removed before reconstruction can begin.

With proper management of arthritis and other rheumatic conditions —both medical and rehabilitative—in the majority of cases a useful, active life can be assured. Because each case has its own particular makeup, however, this management is usually tailored to the individual's needs.

Adherence to the program your doctor has designed for you is vital if he is going to be able to stop the advance of the arthritic condition and reverse the damage which has already been done.

In the succeeding chapters you will be learning about the origins, symptoms, and variations of osteoarthritis, rheumatoid arthritis, gout and related conditions. You will also learn how your doctor can help you feel better, and how you can help yourself.

CHAPTER 2

Osteoarthritis -- *"The Wear and Tear Disease"*

"Osteoarthritis is man's oldest and most common disease. Beginning at least with the dinosaurs, almost every animal that can walk has been susceptible to arthritis. As a human affliction, it is certain that every person over 60 could be found to have it to some degree. Only a small percentage of those with osteoarthritis have it badly enough to notice it, but when it is troublesome something has to be done about it and proper medical treatment is necessary."

So stated Dr. William E. Reynolds, Director of Medical and Scientific Affairs for the U.S. Arthritis Foundation.

Your osteoarthritis is troublesome enough to seek a doctor's care or you wouldn't be reading this book. And there are at least 10 million others like you who need the relief and management that only a doctor can provide.

This disease plays no favorites. Just about as many women as men are affected. However there is a differentiation according to age. For those under 45 the ratio of male to female sufferers is two to one. Up the age gap to between 55 and 65 and the females take the lead. After age 65 the ratio becomes equal.

Osteoarthritis is a disease of the joints which involves a breakdown of cartilage and other tissues which make it possible for a joint to operate normally. Inflammation may or may not be present, but it is usually minimal and not of primary concern. Because this disease is more common in older adults it is often described as "degenerative joint disease." It may also be referred to as hypertrophic arthritis, senescent arthritis, or arthrosis as it is more commonly known in Europe.

Evidence of this disease has been found in the skeletal remains of Neanderthal man, who roamed the earth 42,000 years ago. It has also been seen in the fossil remains of dinosaurs from the Mesozoic Period, some 200 million years ago. Needless to say, it is no stranger to the planet earth!

Arthritis per se has many forms, including rheumatoid arthritis, which we will be discussing in the next chapter. Ankylosing spondylitis, rheumatic fever, and gout, among many other forms, also fall into the general category of the rheumatic diseases. Each of these is a distinct and separate illness with different effects on the patient.

Don't confuse osteoarthritis with rheumatoid arthritis because there are very distinct differences. Rheumatoid arthritis always involves inflammation of the joints and can affect the entire body's system. In osteoarthritis the problem is localized and inflammation is due only to irritation of the joint lining.

WHAT MAKES YOUR JOINTS MOVE?

The human body is remarkable in many ways, and one of the body's supreme achievements is the movability of the joints. What allows them to move? Cartilage, ligaments, and lubrication.

If you were to examine a human skeleton you would see that the bones in each joint are shaped so that they fit together. In the living human being, the ends of the joint bones are covered with cartilage which has the quality of smooth, rubbery gristle. This acts as an elastic cushion; but it has to be lubricated to permit smooth movement between the bones.

The joint ends are kept together by sheets and strands of dense fibers. These are called ligaments, and they completely enclose the joints in a capsule-like arrangement. This capsule, in turn, has a lining called the synovial membrane. This is the source of lubrication for your joints. The synovial membrane secretes a slippery fluid which makes it possible for the joints to operate smoothly.

When osteoarthritis begins its damaging ways the first thing that happens is a softening, pitting, and fraying of the smooth cartilage surface. These conditions in themselves pave the way for further damage

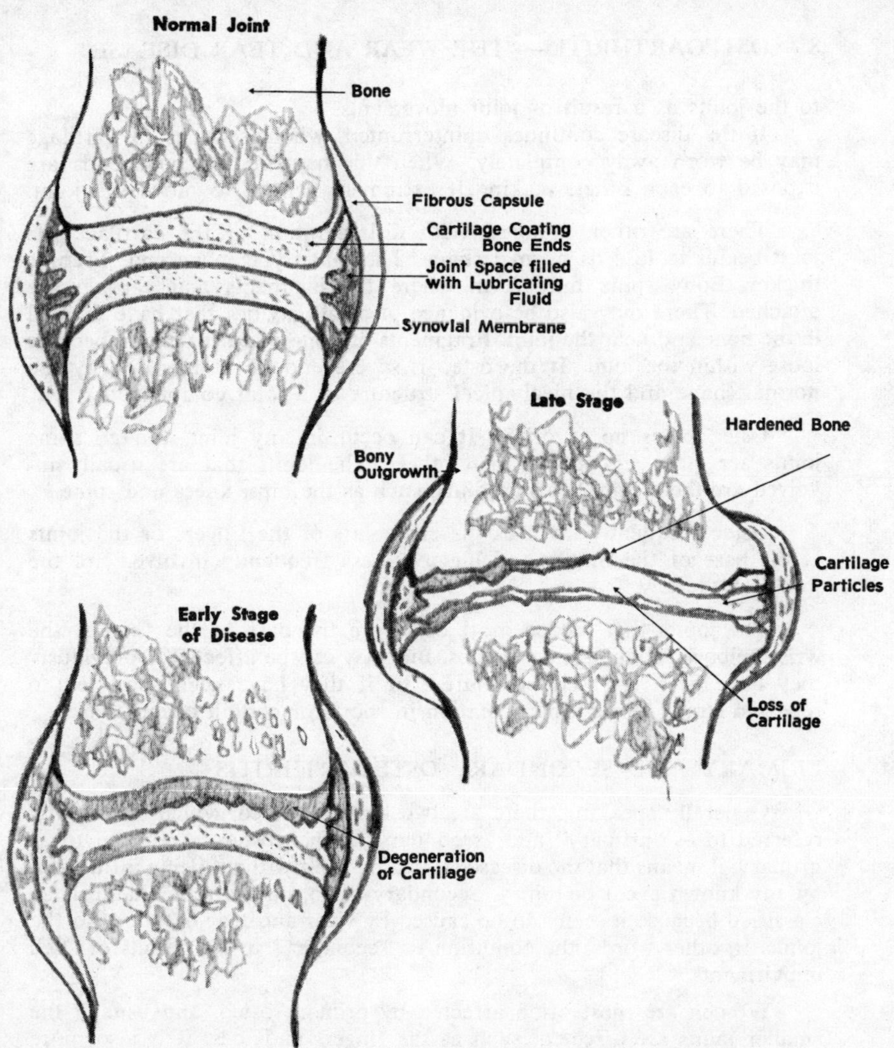

Drawing above shows (1) a joint as it appears normally before the deterioration of arthritis begins; (2) the joint in the early stages of arthritis, with degeneration of cartilage; and (3) an arthritic joint in a late stage of the disease, with characteristic bony outgrowth, hardened bone, cartilage particles, and loss of cartilage.

to the joints as a result of joint movements.

If the disease continues uninterrupted, whole sections of cartilage may be worn away completely. When this happens the bone ends are exposed to each other, making it extremely painful to move the joint.

There are other changes. With disintegration of the cartilage the joint begins to lose its normal shape. The underlying bone ends become thicker. Bony spurs may form where the ligaments and capsule are attached. There may also be evidence of small cavities that have formed in the bone end near the joint. Fragments of bone or cartilage can become loose within the joint. If the osteo is severe enough it may destroy the normal shape and the mechanical structure of a joint completely.

Osteo plays no favorites. It can occur in any joint, though some joints are more susceptible than others. The joints that are usually involved are the weight-bearing joints, such as the hips, knees and spine.

Osteo frequently involves the end joints of the fingers or the joints at the base of the thumb and big toe. Less frequently involved are the joints of the jaw.

The joints that escape most often are the base of the fingers, the wrists, elbows, shoulders, or ankles. But they can be affected if previously they have been diseased or injured, or if they have been subjected to repeated strain through participation in sports or certain occupations.

PRIMARY AND SECONDARY OSTEOARTHRITIS

Generally speaking, there are two kinds of osteo, which are usually referred to as "primary" and "secondary." When osteo is referred to as primary, it means that the disease started by itself without being influenced by any known event or injury. Secondary osteo, on the other hand, is so classified because it seems to be caused by wear and tear or injury to the joints. In other words, the condition is "secondary" to the results of such impairments.

Women are most often affected by primary osteo, and usually the smaller joints are affected, such as the fingers and toes. It is also more generalized and occurs earlier in life, sometimes in the late thirties or early forties. In these cases there is frequently a strong family history of osteo.

Secondary osteo, on the other hand, tends to affect the larger joints and usually occurs later in life. Small joints may also be affected, however, if they have been exposed to abnormal strain. Secondary osteo can also occur earlier in life if a particular joint has been seriously injured.

You can have two kinds of arthritis or "mixed arthritis," such as rheumatoid arthritis and osteoarthritis, at the same time. This is usually caused by rheumatoid arthritis. When joints become chronically inflamed, as in rheumatoid arthritis, this can lead to the development of secondary osteoarthritis.

The Arthritis Foundation has this to say about occupations that may lead to osteoarthritis: "The pattern in which joints are affected is often related to the particular stress and strain of a particular occupation. A baseball pitcher is more likely to develop osteoarthritis in his throwing arm, especially in the elbow. A football player may get osteoarthritis in his knees. Ballet dancers have been known to get osteoarthritis of the ankles. These are examples of the 'wearing out' of specific joint tissues by excessive use."

WHAT CAUSES OSTEOARTHRITIS?

No one knows what causes osteoarthritis, though there are many existing theories. Some doctors believe heredity may be the most important factor, especially in primary osteo. On the other hand, heredity may not be a factor in secondary osteo. A joint may succumb to the disease only because it has had more strain than it could bear. It can also be caused by being overweight which, in itself, places unusual strain on the weight-bearing joints.

Many of the handicaps associated with osteoarthritis are not necessarily the result of joint disturbances. Very often they are the result of muscle weakness due to lack of exercise or use and/or "bad habits" such as slouching, stooping over while walking, sitting on very low and very soft chairs or sofas or on poorly designed or adjusted automobile seats.

In fact, many of the discomforts associated with osteoarthritis may be due to today's sedentary way of life. How many people walk when they can ride, even though the destination is near at hand, such as a neighborhood store? Today many people sit for long periods watching television in poorly designed and constructed chairs and sofas.

There is also a tendency toward overweight. Many cases of osteoarthritis from the waist down seen in females past the age of 40 are due to abnormal joint strain caused by obesity. Another factor is the choice of footwear, especially in women. The combination of poor footwear and obesity creates an improper gait and improper distribution of weight, which in turn causes arthritic changes in the knees.

Why do some people get osteoarthritis sooner than others? Why is it that some victims suffer severe osteoarthritis at a comparatively early age while other members of their family may go through life without being bothered hardly at all? The answers to these questions are still unknown and are still the subject of intense, continuing research.

SYMPTOMS

Many people may have osteoarthritis in such a mild form that they don't even realize they have it, even though on examination the doctor would find evidence of the disease. But the more than 10 million known osteo sufferers in Canada and the United States are well aware of the disease and its symptoms.

First and foremost is the pain associated with osteo. This may be a mild aching and soreness in certain joints, especially during movement. Some patients may experience a continuing, nagging pain even when they are at rest.

Probably the second most common symptom is the loss of mobility. The patient is made aware of this when he finds it difficult and painful to perform relatively easy movements of the affected joints. Sometimes there can be a severe loss of motion or inability to move certain joints in a specific way.

These effects take their toll on the surrounding muscle tissues. Because the patient tends to resist mobility of the affected joints, the muscles become weakened through lack of use. This has its effect, too, on body coordination and posture, depending on the joints involved.

There can also be evidence of "referred pain." When this happens, the pain is felt some distance away from the joint which is involved. An example of this is an osteoarthritic hip which produces pain in the area near the patient's knees.

The sources of the pain are irritation and pressure on nerve endings, muscle tension, and muscle fatigue. Every patient reacts individually to these conditions. It is not unusual for a patient with a severely affected joint to have less pain than a patient who only seems to have a comparatively minor problem. In any case the pain is more severe if the joint has been overused or if the joint has had a long period of inactivity.

There are usually no "generalized" symptoms. When your doctor makes this observation he means that there are no symptoms of sickness such as fever or loss of weight. Generally speaking, you "don't feel sick."

HEBERDEN'S AND BOUCHARD'S NODES

Osteo has other common characteristics in its primary form in which women are most often affected. Among these is the incidence of Heberden's nodes or bony enlargements of the end joints of the fingers. These can appear as early as age 40. When the middle joints of the fingers are similarly enlarged these are referred to as Bouchard's nodes.

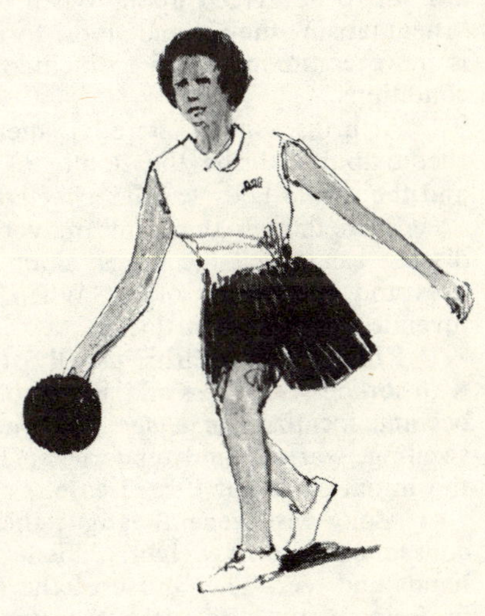

Although these conditions are usually associated with primary osteo, they can also occur in secondary osteo when fingers have been injured. When this happens the condition is sometimes referred to as "baseball finger" or "bowler's finger."

These conditions can be painless; but sometimes they may appear suddenly, with redness, swelling, tenderness and aching. There may also be a numbness and tingling of the fingertips and clumsiness of the hands. In spite of the distress and pain of these conditions, in most cases a good function of the hands can be achieved, and crippling is not likely to occur.

CHAPTER 3

Rheumatoid Arthritis

IF DOCTORS KNEW THE CAUSE, they might be able to find a cure for rheumatoid arthritis, which is probably the most severe and painful of all the rheumatic diseases. Early diagnosis and treatment are essential if doctors are going to be able to prevent the severe crippling associated with rheumatoid arthritis. Research offers promise that in the near future patients will be able to receive a great deal more help in the management of this chronic illness.

"Rheumatism" in itself denotes unspecific or unexplained aches and pains that may occur in joints or muscles or both. A precise definition has yet to be agreed upon. When doctors in Great Britain use the term "rheumatism" they include most forms of arthritis. In this country arthritis is more commonly used to include rheumatism as well as other similar conditions.

Arthritis, quite literally, means "inflammation of a joint." In rheumatoid arthritis the dominant characteristic is joint inflammation, and the whole body can be affected.

Even though the joints may be the primary source of attack, this disease can affect the lungs, skin, blood vessels, muscles, spleen, heart, eyes and almost any organ. When it occurs in children, it is known as juvenile rheumatoid arthritis.

Rheumatoid arthritis usually starts with a feeling of general fatigue, with soreness, stiffness and aching of the joints. Gradually these symptoms become localized in a specific joint or in several joints, causing pain, swelling, warmth and tenderness. The hands are frequently involved in the initial stages of this disease.

Along with general fatigue there is usually a loss of appetite and a consequent loss of weight. Patients frequently complain of cold, sweaty hands and feet. The course of the disease varies in length of attack and in frequency. Quite often the symptoms will gradually disappear, followed by a period of relatively good health, and then a sudden flare up will begin the attack all over again.

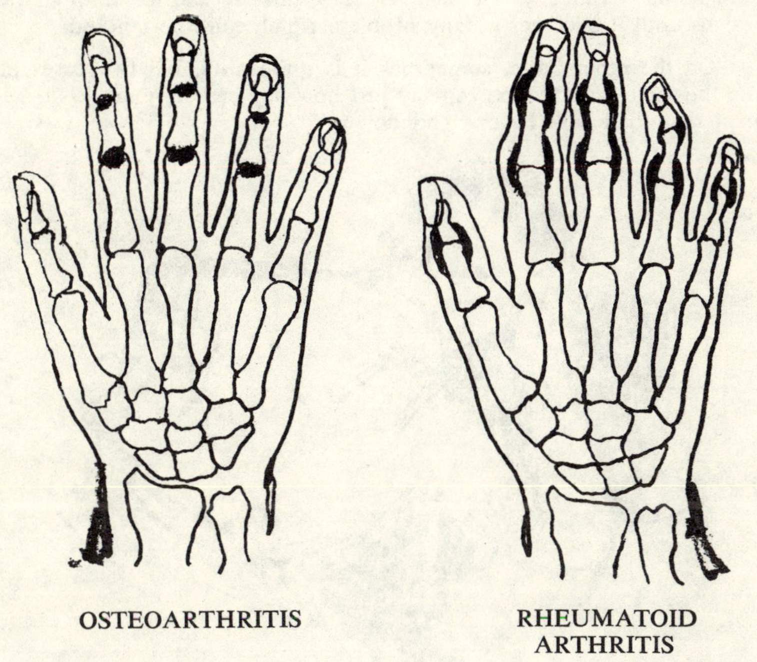

Illustration of hands above show differences between osteoarthritis and rheumatoid arthritis. In osteoarthritis there is a deterioration in the joints without the swelling that usually accompanies rheumatoid arthritis. Also, in rheumatoid arthritis deformities are more likely to occur.

The Arthritis Foundation describes it in this way: "Of all forms of arthritis, rheumatoid arthritis is the most dangerous, destructive and disabling. It can strike suddenly and progress rapidly to an acute and seriously damaging stage. More often it comes on subtly and deceptively. The symptoms appear for a few days and then go away again . . . come back later a little worse, and disappear again . . . and return once more with new violence. There may be weeks or months between goings and comings, but gradually the disease reappears at shorter and shorter intervals until it becomes a daily problem which can't be ignored.

"On the other hand, sometimes it is quite mild. No two cases are quite the same, and no one can say just how any case is going to go . . . except that there will be ups and downs."

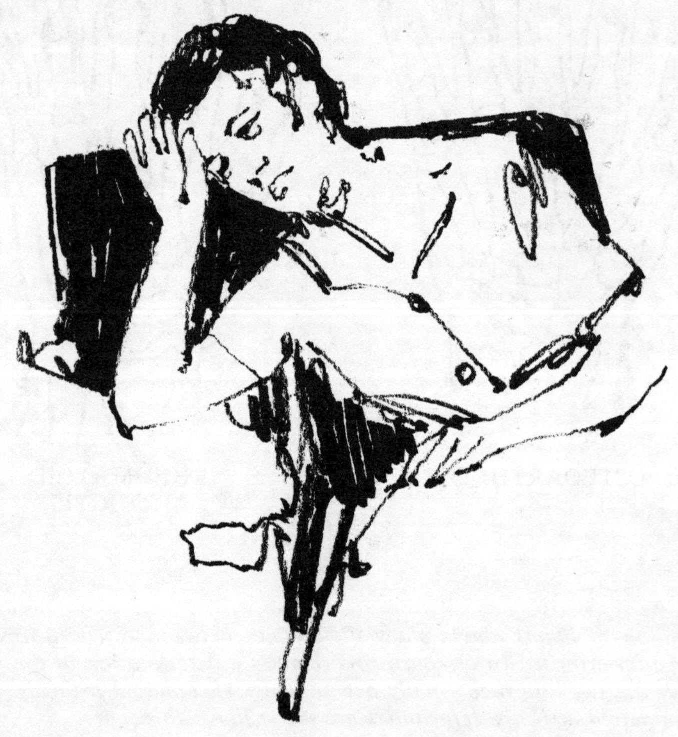

WHEN THERE IS REMISSION

When the doctor says there appears to have been a remission of the disease, he means that the disease appears to have gone away by itself. In the case of rheumatoid arthritis, the pain, stiffness and swelling, even in severe cases, may suddenly stop and not return for months or even years. It may never come back. This happens in about one out of five or six cases.

But the patient should never become overly optimistic about his condition. Damage has already been done, and this will not vanish. Out of sight, out of mind. You may not be aware of this, but your doctor is.

Rheumatoid arthritis sufferers, though only aware of pain in certain joints, must realize that their whole body is affected by this disease. The primary sources of attack are the hands, arms, hips, legs and feet. This disease also attacks the body's connective tissue.

Patients tire easily. Their appetite is poor. They lose weight and suffer from anemia. It is not uncommon for the lymph glands and spleen to become enlarged. Fever is commonly seen in juvenile rheumatoid arthritis.

The affected joints become stiff, then they swell and become tender and painful. This makes full motion difficult. These conditions are worse at the beginning of the day, when the patient first gets up. Then they improve after he has been up and moving for awhile. Some patients develop small lumps under the skin—usually at the elbows, knees, and ankles. These are called rheumatoid nodules.

WHAT CAUSES THE CRIPPLING

Inflammation is the most common characteristic of rheumatoid arthritis. And it is the inflammation, if left unchecked or untreated, which can lead to crippling.

Inflammation begins in the area where the joints meet, which is enclosed in the capsule that contains the lubricating fluid. The inner layer of the capsule, the synovial membrane, is the beginning point of the inflammation. As the inflammation continues, this membrane begins to swell, causing the inflammation to spread to the cartilage connected to the end bones of the joint. In time the cartilage may be destroyed so that the joint may become fused. When this happens the joint becomes rigid and immovable. At other times, the bone endings, uncovered by cartilage, cause severe pain with motion.

This destruction of the joint is a slow but continuing process, if left untreated. And as the destruction of the joint continues, contractions develop which can cause deformities. If these deformities are severe enough they can cause crippling. One example of this, and a common one, is misshapen fingers. The fingers become drawn back and sideways. In this crooked condition they become practically useless for the normal functions for which they were intended.

CRIPPLING CAN BE PREVENTED

Crippling can occur, but in most cases it can be prevented. Unfortunately too many rheumatoid arthritis sufferers (from 20% to 40% according to a report from the American Rheumatism Association) never seek medical help. If inflammatory activity continues over a period of years without treatment, the chances of the sufferer developing crippling deformities are that much greater than for the patient under a doctor's care.

According to the ARA Report, "The dramatic appearance of the severely crippled patient with rheumatoid arthritis, a common sight in clinic waiting rooms, tends to exaggerate the gravity of this disease in the minds of fellow patients and physicians. Even among the patients requiring hospitalization, prolonged followup reveals one quarter are able to carry on their usual activities completely, one third severely crippled, and the remainder with mild degrees of incapacitation. About 10% of the hospital-treated patients become bed or wheelchair bound."

It should be stated that those who have severe attacks in the initial stages of this disease may fare better than those who suffer from continuing but relatively mild attacks. One reason for this may be that those suffering great pain in an acute attack receive heavy doses of medication and treatment which ultimately have a beneficial and long-lasting effect. Those who have mild complaints tend to require milder treatment, if they seek a doctor's care. But, as is too often the case, they do not seek a doctor's care soon enough or often enough. Too many people with rheumatoid arthritis are content to suffer mild aches and pains or stiffness without complaint, not realizing how serious their condition is and that it can lead to crippling deformities.

Many physicians refer to rheumatoid arthritis as a particularly demanding disease from their point of view as well as their patients. Those who suffer from rheumatoid arthritis must have the patience to accept long-term treatment; and physicians who treat them must be prepared to manage the disease over a long period of time. Too many patients are content with "undertreatment," seeking help only when the disease flares up.

As George E. Ehrlich, M.D., associate professor of rehabilitation medicine at Temple University School of Medicine has stated, "Crisis therapy is just not good enough. The patient needs total care—a program of constant supervision from the moment his disease is identified."

CHAPTER 4

Gout

"Gout is generally thought to be a rather comical disease, and artists both ancient and modern have made fun of its victims. It is rather difficult to know why this has been so, since it is one of the most painful of all diseases, and by attacking the heart and the kidneys may eventually lead to death if it is not checked."

So wrote Dr. W. S. C. Copeman, one of England's leading rheumatologists, in 1967. He later went on to explain that new medications now made this disease much less of a threat to the sufferer. This will be discussed in full in the chapter on "Treatment by Medication."

Gout or gouty arthritis is one of the major arthritic diseases. It has very specific differences in cause and effect. Gout essentially is a disease which affects the joints and the kidneys. This is caused by abnormal body chemistries which cause an excess amount of uric acid.

Acute attacks of gout are caused by the formation of crystals of monosodium urate, a uric acid salt, in one or more joints. When this happens inflammation and pain follow. Usually the joints affected in a gout attack are more painful than a swollen joint in rheumatoid arthritis or osteoarthritis. The reason for this is that the inflammation is usually more severe, and this in itself is painful. The severe inflammation is accompanied by physical pressure and chemical irritation of the sensitive nerve endings in the area around the affected joints.

The swelling in the joint area may be more noticeable than in attacks of other forms of arthritis. In any instance of inflammation the blood vessels in the affected area tend to become more porous. They "leak" blood in the affected area, surrounding it with "repair" cells which attempt to take care of the damage but actually cause more swelling. The swelling in itself adds considerably to the pain. Acute attacks of gout can be related to one of a number of causes and are sometimes very difficult to pinpoint.

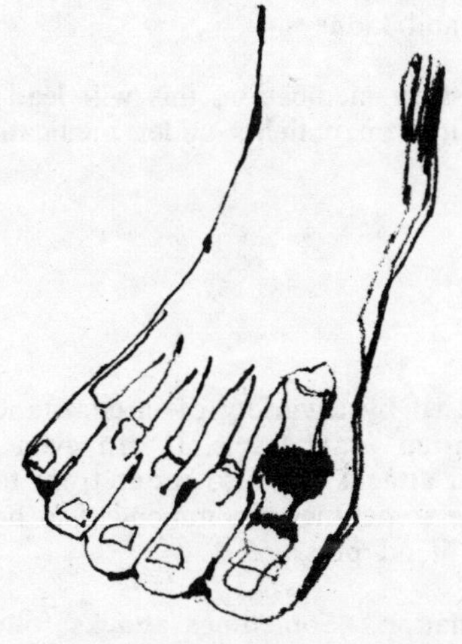

An inside look at a big toe affected by gout.

Every human being's body manufactures uric acid from substances called "purines" in a series of chemical reactions which are quite complex. Many common, everyday foods also contain high amounts of purine. These should be avoided by the gout sufferer. Among foods with high purine content are anchovies, sardines, and animal organs such as sweetbreads, brains, kidney and liver. Among beverages, beer contains a high amount of purine. These and other foods and beverages which should be avoided by the gout sufferer are described in detail in the chapter on "The Importance of Diet."

HOW THE BODY RIDS ITSELF OF URIC ACID

The body acts in several ways to rid itself of uric acid. It can be voided through urination or through the intestinal tract or even through perspiration. Many physicians believe that in some patients with gout the normal mechanisms to eliminate uric acid through the kidneys are impaired, thus causing the excess amounts in the body. This is in contrast to those cases in which the excess uric acid is due to overproduction.

According to current research some gout sufferers have both these strikes against them. The end result is that uric acid crystals tend to collect in tissues such as joints, skin and kidneys.

Unless the patient takes the necessary medication, this will lead to acute and chronic attacks of gout. But even patients under medication can have acute attacks.

ACUTE ATTACKS OF GOUT

Acute attacks of gout can be caused by a variety of circumstances which result in a rapid increase in serum urate levels. It can even be caused by injury to a gouty joint. Gout attacks can also result from taking thiozides or "water pills," which are sometimes recommended to help reduce weight or bring relief to high blood pressure.

According to the Arthritis Foundation, "Sometimes attacks follow injections of drugs. People with gout quite frequently suffer attacks after surgical operations. In fact, an acute attack of arthritis following a surgical operation always raises a suspicion of gout. Patients who have gout should always advise the surgeon of this fact if an operation is being planned."

High living, in itself, is not a cause of gout. Rich foods, taken in moderation, as well as alcoholic beverages when not drunk to excess, will not necessarily cause attacks of gout. As in all diseases, there is a great variation in the severity of the condition from individual to individual. This is as true in gout as it is in any other disease.

Many gout patients may need some dietary controls. Most patients, however, have no significant restrictions as long as they remain under medication.

In many cases the person susceptible to attacks of gout is likely to know his own intolerances in regard to food and drink. He should be extremely careful in avoiding the foods or beverages which can trigger an attack of gout.

INCIDENCE OF TOPHACEOUS GOUT

In some gout conditions, tophi, which are deposits of monosodium urate monohydrate, a white chalky compound of uric acid, gradually accumulate in the tissues. When this condition exists physicians refer to it as "tophaceous gout."

The tophi generally collect in tissues near the joints and are sometimes seen near the elbows or near the rims of the ears. Nonarticular tophi (not related to a joint) are usually painless, but when the mass of tophi grows in a joint it can lead to impediment of joint motion and cause pain. Sometimes tophi that collect in the ears become quite hard and take on a lumplike quality.

In most cases, however, tophi form only after a person has had gout for a long time without proper treatment.

GOUT AND KIDNEY DISEASE

Gout in many patients may lead to problems in the function of the kidney, since this is one of the prime areas in which urate deposits accumulate. This can cause impairment of kidney function and a scarring of kidney tissues. It may also lead to formation of kidney stones.

Kidney stones caused by gout are quite similar to other kidney stones; however, unlike other kidney stones they don't cast a shadow when the kidney is x-rayed. So instead of using the x-ray test, certain diagnostic dyes are injected. If the dyes are not excreted by the kidney, then it may be assumed that the gouty kidney stones are causing a blockage.

The amount of pain involved will depend on the size as well as the location of the stones. Sometimes they will pass through the kidney of their own accord. But when they cause blockage then surgery may be required to correct this condition. According to some authorities the number of gout patients who develop kidney stones is not high.

Kidney stones, however, are at least twenty times more frequent in gouty patients than in those without gout.

The Committee of the American Rheumatism Association's report on gout expressed a generally good prognosis for gout and pointed to several studies which indicate that there is no significant decrease in life expectancy. Declared the committee, "The outlook is less favorable for the patient who develops the disease at an early age, but even here there is reason to hope that intelligent treatment conscientiously carried out will result in normal longevity."

GOUT AS A FAMILY TRAIT

It is generally believed that gout does tend to run in families. The chemical defects which cause the body to produce too much uric acid or do not permit the body to get rid of uric acid fast enough are hereditary factors which can be passed on to the children from either the mother or the father. Yet it is not necessarily to be expected that if either parent has gout he or she will pass it on to their children. It can happen, but it doesn't have to happen.

Gout attacks in children are very rare, but when they do happen the child should receive treatment immediately to prevent any crippling effects.

Gout is also a rare disease for women before menopause, occurring in only about five percent of the cases reported. This may be due to the fact that women usually have lower average blood uric acid levels than men. If a gout attack does occur in women it is usually after the menopause.

Men are the major sufferers from gout. Its onset can occur anytime after puberty.

FREQUENCY OF ATTACKS

In the usual course of this disease there may be a lapse of several years between the first and second acute attacks. But then the attacks are likely to become more frequent, occurring as often as six times a year. They may also become more severe, lasting for several weeks and involving several joints.

One of the classic descriptions of an acute attack of gout was written by Thomas Sydenham, a 17th century English physician, who described it thus:

"The victim goes to bed and sleeps in good health. About two o'clock in the morning he is awakened by a severe pain in the great toe; more rarely in the heel, ankle or instep. This pain is like that of a dislocation, and yet the parts feel as if cold water were poured over them. Then follow chills and shivers, and a little fever.

"The pain, which was at first moderate, becomes more intense. With its intensity, the chills and shivers increase. After a time this comes to its height, accommodating itself to the bones and ligaments of tarsus and metatarsus.

"Now it is a violent stretching and tearing of the ligaments—now it is a gnawing pain and now a pressure and tightening. So exquisite and lively meanwhile is the feeling of the part affected, that it cannot bear the weight of the bedcloths nor the jar of a person walking in the room."

This is a rather discouraging description of what the gout sufferer had to look forward to in the 17th century. Fortunately, medical science has made dramatic progress in recent years in developing medication which has brought long-sought relief to the gout sufferer and which helps prevent acute attacks.

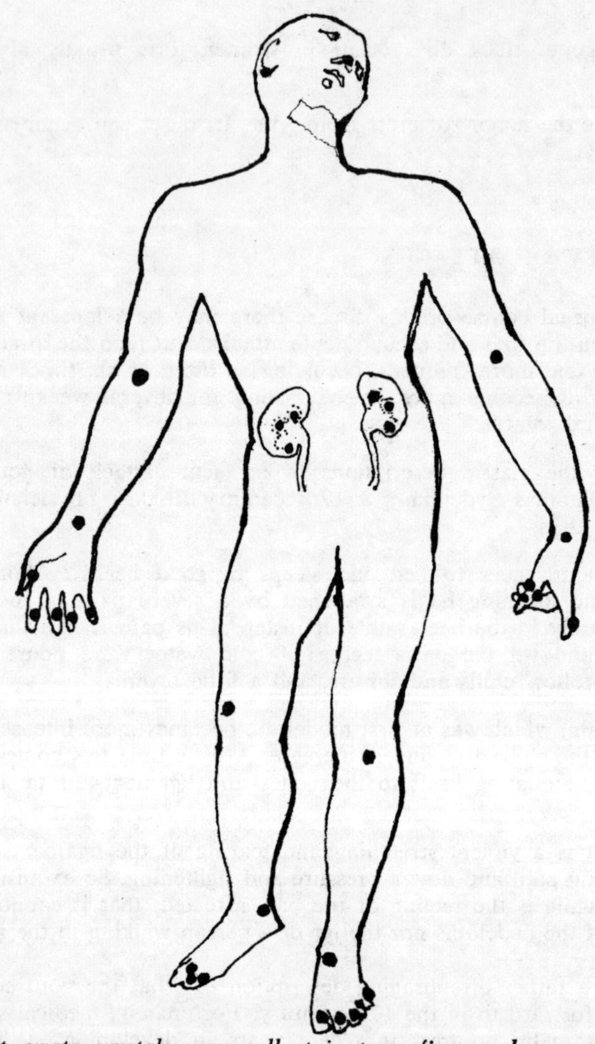

In gout, urate crystals may collect in toes, fingers, knees, and elbows, even on the tips of the ear and nose. The gout prone areas are indicated by dots in the above drawing.

CHAPTER 5

Juvenile Rheumatoid Arthritis and Rheumatic Fever

The number of children who suffer from rheumatoid arthritis is relatively small when you consider the millions of adults who suffer from this disease. But when it does strike a child every precaution should be taken, including immediate treatment from a qualified physician.

When rheumatoid arthritis develops in a child, the joint symptoms may be much milder than in adults and occasionally absent. These children may appear very ill, however, with high fever and skin rashes that suggest an infectious disease. In other cases, and especially in older children, the onset of the disease may resemble more closely the symptoms seen in the adult form of rheumatoid arthritis.

In addition to the fact that juvenile rheumatoid arthritis may continue into adulthood, parents should keep in mind that this disease, in spite of the mild form it may appear to take, is just as serious as adult rheumatoid arthritis. Even though the pain may be localized in one or more joints, the disease is affecting the whole body.

Some forms of juvenile rheumatoid arthritis may affect the eyes to the point of causing blindness. This is a complication which should be very carefully watched and treated.

The affected joints should be handled with a great deal of care. They should be kept in proper alignment so as to prevent any unnecessary deformities. Once the child has recovered from an acute attack it may be necessary to limit his activities in games and sports so he will not injure any of the joints that have been affected and thus bring on another attack.

The Arthritis Foundation offers the following advice to parents with children who have rheumatoid arthritis: "Despite the fact that there is now no specific cure for juvenile rheumatoid arthritis, children can be greatly helped by proper care and treatment that must be under a physician's continued supervision. This includes the use of antirheumatic drugs as well as physical therapy. Chances of overcoming permanent crippling or other consequences are excellent, providing that the young patient receives prompt medical care.

"By being alert to the disease, by understanding its nature and the manner of its treatment, parents who maintain continuous care and give unflagging love and reassurance to an afflicted child play a key role in brightening the outlook for successful treatment."

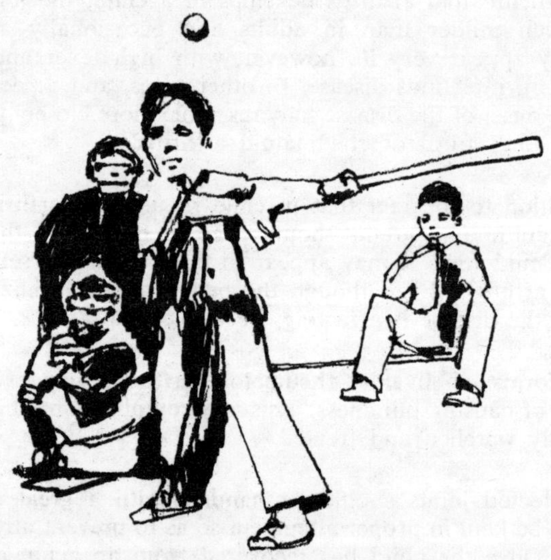

Children who have recovered from an acute attack of rheumatoid arthritis may have to avoid games and sports that might lead to injury of any of the joints that have been affected and thus bring on another attack.

RHEUMATIC FEVER

Rheumatic fever has long been known to be caused by a streptococcus infection. The chief danger in this disease is the potential damage to the heart. It is also a disease that tends to recur.

It is considered an arthritic disease because it causes an inflammation of the joints. Although the arthritis symptoms are painful, they can usually be controlled and eventually disappear.

Parents should keep in mind the fact that even though a streptococcus infection is always associated with rheumatic fever and can cause a recurrence of the disease, only a small percentage of children with streptococcal sore throat develop rheumatic fever.

This disease can occur at any age. It is rare in infancy, but it is most common between the ages of five and 15 years.

The severity of a rheumatic fever attack is directly related to the severity of the streptococcus infection. If administered in time, antibiotics can stop the disease in its tracks. But if it is left to linger the streptococcus infection can trigger an acute attack of rheumatic fever.

According to the American Rheumatism Association, from 10% to 50% of patients who have had previous attacks of rheumatic fever will have a recurrence following a streptococcal infection. The tendency to a recurrence, however, becomes less with each passing year.

Thanks to advances in antibiotics, such as penicillin and other forms of antimicrobial therapy, the incidence of rheumatic fever has declined. Rheumatic fever, however, is still one of the most serious diseases affecting children. Parents should be particularly vigilant whenever there is an outbreak of streptococcus infection.

HOW THE DISEASE ATTACKS THE BODY

As in rheumatoid arthritis, the entire body is affected by rheumatic fever. But the greatest danger lies in the effect it may have on the heart. All areas of the heart can be affected. This includes the membrane that lines the cavities of the heart, the heart muscle itself, the membraneous sac that encloses the heart, and the heart's valves. Enlargement of the heart due to the inflammation can leave permanent scars in the heart or its valves which cause permanent damage.

As the disease progresses, the fever tends to remain high. This is accompanied by arthritic symptoms. Most often affected are the joints of the extremities. But all joints can be affected.

The pain and swelling in one joint may subside, but then the arthritis "migrates" to other joints over a period of days or weeks. The first sign that the heart may have been affected is in the detection of heart murmurs.

A characteristic rash is also common to rheumatic fever. This is not always noticeable but is usually evident after the patient has had a warm bath. It can appear almost anywhere, but is usually evident either on the back, chest, stomach, hands or feet.

The acute inflammation associated with rheumatic fever usually subsides in about six weeks; but it can persist for as long as three months. When the inflammation leaves, the affected parts of the body, including the heart, begin to heal and may heal completely. The danger in rheumatic fever is that scarring of the heart valves can cause serious problems when the patient reaches adulthood.

Before the advent of miracle drugs such as the antibiotics, most rheumatic fever patients could expect the disease to reoccur, increasing the possibility of permanent heart damage. But this is no longer true. If the patient survives the initial attack without damage to his heart, the chances are that with proper treatment he will escape the permanent effects of rheumatic heart disease.

Once the disease is in process, certain measures can be taken to minimize permanent damage to the heart; however, these are not always successful.

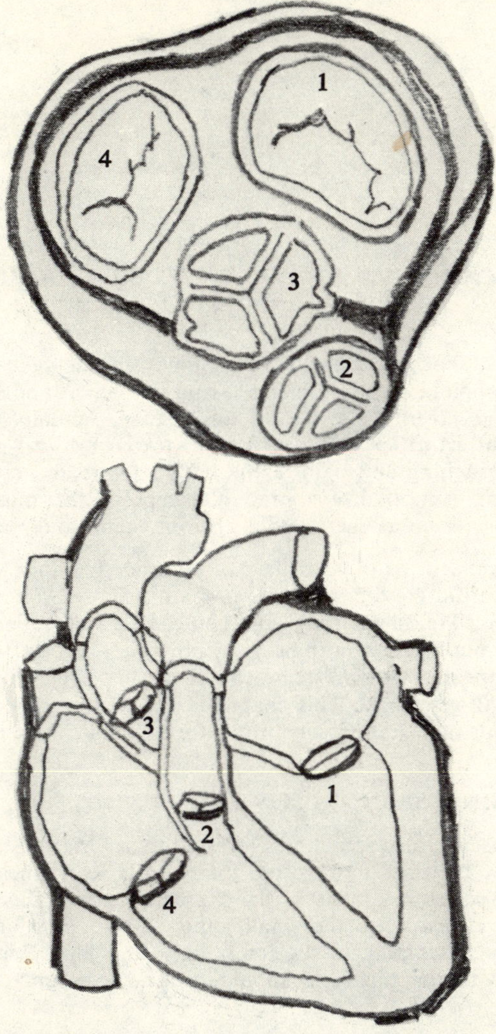

Shown in the drawing above is the top view of the heart with the valves identified by number. Below is a side view of the heart and corresponding valves. In rheumatic fever, it is the scarring of the valves which can lead to serious problems when the child reaches adulthood.

CHAPTER 6

Other Forms of Arthritis or Rheumatism

Because arthritis or rheumatism can take so many forms, this has compounded the problems facing physicians and scientists in their attempts to discover the causes of this disease. Actually there are almost 100 different arthritic conditions known to the medical profession, all of which cause aching and pain in the body's joints and connective tissues. Inflammation is not always present except in the most serious forms of the disease, such as rheumatoid arthritis, gout, and rheumatic fever.

All major forms of arthritis are chronic. In other words, once you have an arthritic condition, be it common or rare, you will probably always have it. Treatment may give you the desired relief from pain and discomfort, but there is nothing your physician can do to make the condition disappear. Without treatment, however, it is very likely that the condition will get worse. This chapter will describe some of the less common (though none the less painful) forms of arthritis and rheumatism.

ANKYLOSING SPONDYLITIS

This disease, also sometimes referred to as "Marie-Strumpell disease," attacks men 10 times more often than it attacks women. It is a disease of the spine which has many of the characteristics of rheumatoid arthritis. First to be affected are the small joints of the spine and the sacroiliac joints. This causes pain in the lower back and legs. Eventually the pain may spread to the hips and shoulders. The eyes may also become inflamed.

Back discomfort is usually the first symptom. Rest brings no relief. The initial attack may be very acute, but like other arthritic diseases, ankylosing spondylitis is usually insidious, with intermittent episodes of pain in the lower back and hips. The pain can be very intense, particularly when certain movements are made.

Morning stiffness in the back is usually noticeable. Quite often the patient may be awakened early in the morning by pain. By walking about he can achieve some measure of relief. The pain associated with this disease tends to grow progressively worse and leads to restricted motion of the back. Sometimes the development of limited back movement may have no apparent pain associated with it.

The stiffness of the spine in this disease may eventually progress until the spine is completely rigid. Another characteristic is the development of a curvature of the spine which forces the patient into a stooped position, sometimes referred to as "poker back."

No one yet knows the cause of this disease. The theory that heredity plays a part in the incidence of ankylosing spondylitis is generally accepted.

The disease usually begins when the patient is in his late teens and seldom begins after age 30. Immediate treatment is essential if the discomfort and deformity associated with this disease are to be controlled. After several years the disease usually comes to an end, but the stiffness and deformity lingers on. The pain, however, is usually minor at this point.

SYSTEMUS LUPUS ERYTHEMATOSUS (SLE)

In contrast to ankylosing spondylitis, SLE or systemic lupus erythematosus is a disease that primarily affects young women of childbearing age rather than men. This disease involves inflammation and damage to the connective tissues throughout the body. The skin, the internal organs, and the joints are affected, with the pain of arthritis one of the dominant conditions.

This disease may have a variety of symptoms, including fever, skin rash, loss of weight, a general feeling of weakness and fatigue, and anemia as well as joint pains. Kidney problems may develop and the nervous system may be affected.

It does not follow a regular course. The SLE sufferer, like the patient with other forms of arthritis, will have her ups and downs. Many of the symptoms will suddenly stop and the patient may appear to be improving. Then the disease will return with a sudden flare-up. There is no sure cure as yet for this disease, and treatment usually involves medication in an attempt to alter the course of the disease.

SCLERODERMA

Another rare form of arthritis that affects the body's connective tissue is scleroderma. This disease causes a thickening and hardening of the skin, giving it a leather-like quality. Inflammation is sometimes involved as well as a scarring of the muscles and internal organs. Like SLE, scleroderma affects more women than men. It can begin at any age but it usually starts when the patient is in her forties or fifties.

It can advance rapidly, or it can stop and start again, as in other forms of arthritis. One prominent rheumatologist, John J. Calabro, M.D., has described scleroderma "as if the hardening of the arteries to which all aging humans are subject stiffens the body's largest organ, the skin. That is the way of scleroderma, whose name derives from the Greek *skleros* (hard) and *derma* (skin). But as in so many other rheumatic disorders, the name is misleading.

"The disorder is more accurately described by the more all-inclusive term 'progressive systemic sclerosis.' It is a rare, relentless systemic disorder of connective tissue. The process of sclerosis primarily affects the elasticity of the skin, the joints, and, often with serious consequences, the kidneys, lungs, and heart."

PSORIATIC ARTHRITIS

One of the most common skin diseases is psoriasis, which is known to affect more than four million people in the United States and Canada. According to the Arthritis Foundation, about one out of every 10 cases of psoriasis is complicated by arthritis which has the characteristics of rheumatoid arthritis. In most cases the psoriatic patient may have had the skin disease for many years before he develops arthritis. But occasionally the arthritis develops first, with the fingers and toes usually affected.

Patients with psoriatic arthritis may benefit by some of the same treatment given to patients with rheumatoid arthritis. Physicians, however, have to exercise a great deal of caution to avoid any adverse skin reactions to medication they may prescribe. Control of the skin lesions is of paramount importance in improving the arthritis.

BURSITIS

In most cases of bursitis the shoulder is affected; but bursitis can also occur in other joints such as the hips and elbows. The term "bursitis" comes from the bursa or small sac containing fluid which acts as a buffer or cushioning device between adjoining tissues within a joint structure. When a bursa becomes inflamed, either due to unusual pressure or injury, the result can be extreme tenderness and pain. If the pain is extremely severe, sometimes a physician will inject an anti-inflammatory agent directly into the area producing the greatest pain.

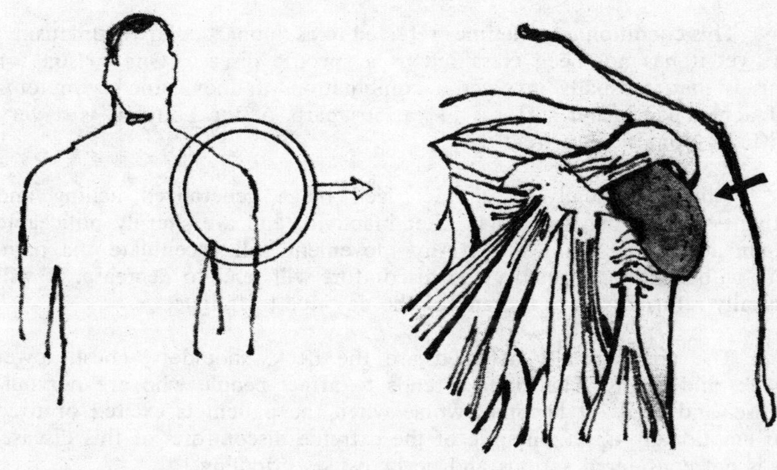

The shoulder is a common site for bursitis. The circled area in the drawing at left is shown in detail in the drawing at right. The shaded area (arrow indicated) is the bursa or site of bursitis. When the bursa becomes inflamed, any movement in the area can cause pain.

REITER'S SYNDROME

This rare form of arthritis is a "three-in-one" disease. It involves *urethritis,* an inflammation of the urethra, the passage through which urine is discharged from the bladder; *conjunctivitis,* an inflammation of the delicate membrane that lines the eyelids; as well as *arthritis* in multiple large joints, most often the knees and ankles. Skin lesions in the penis and diarrhea are also common symptoms. It usually affects young adult males and is very rare in women or children. The disease is usually self-limiting, lasting from six weeks to six months. In about half of the patients recurrences may follow the initial attack, and this can result in deformity of one or more joints.

FIBROSITIS

This condition is sometimes referred to as "nonarticular rheumatism." As yet it has not been classified as a specific disease. One reason for this is that it usually involves a combination of unexplained symptoms of aches, pains, and stiffness in various parts of the body. It is a very difficult condition to treat.

Fibrositis usually is characterized by a generalized aching and stiffness which become worse after inactivity and are sharply noticeable upon awakening from sleep. Any movement will accentuate the pain, but with continued activity the discomfort will tend to decrease. It will usually return again at the end of the day due to fatigue.

The areas usually affected are the neck, shoulders, chest, lower back, and thighs. This disease tends to affect people who are nervous, tense, and weak. It becomes worse when the patient is excited or tired or emotionally upset. In spite of the extreme discomforts of this disease, it is not considered serious and never causes crippling.

ARTHRITIS CAUSED BY INFECTION

Acute or chronic arthritis can be caused when bacteria invade the joints. Examples of this include the incidence of arthritis which develops in patients with tuberculosis, meningitis, and venereal disease. For example, it has been reported that in about one out of every 25 cases of tuberculosis the infection spreads from the lungs to one or more joints, causing arthritis. However, once a physician has determined that the arthritis has been caused by an infection he can obtain beneficial results by using antibiotics.

More than in any other form of arthritis, prompt treatment is necessary in order to avoid any permanent damage to the joints involved.

GERMAN MEASLES SYNDROME

Another type of arthritic condition is the joint pain syndrome of German measles. This condition mainly affects young adults and may, at the beginning, seem to be an attack of rheumatoid arthritis. But the rash, gland swelling and other components distinguish this from the possibility of being rheumatoid arthritis.

At the present time a similar condition has been noted after vaccination for German measles. This can occur shortly after the vaccination or be delayed for a month or two. This condition may last for several weeks to several months. Usually it is amenable to aspirin. Once the condition is cleared it is quite unlikely to reoccur.

ARTHRITIC REACTION TO ALLERGIES

Still another type of arthritic condition is caused by allergic reaction. It is frequently seen as a reaction to anti-Tetanus serum, injected to prevent lockjaw. This condition can result in markedly swollen joints in any part of the body. It is very often indistinguishable from other types of rheumatism or arthritis. The history is the distinguishing factor. This condition usually responds quite readily to corticosteroids used along with antihistamines to counteract the allergen creating condition.

CHAPTER 7

Treatment by Medication

YOUR DOCTOR HAS MANY DRUGS to select from in his treatment of your arthritic condition, whether it be osteoarthritis, rheumatoid arthritis, gout, or one of the rarer forms of arthritis. One of the most commonly used drugs is aspirin.

Because this drug is so widely used for such minor ailments as simple headache and the common cold, many people do not realize how important it can be in the treatment of arthritis. In fact, when someone with arthritis first sees a physician he may be disappointed to learn that his doctor wants him to take aspirin, a drug so common that it can be purchased without a prescription!

WHY ASPIRIN IS SO EFFECTIVE

Most people know that aspirin is used to relieve pain. They also know it can be very effective as a mild sedative. But aspirin is also highly useful in reducing the inflammation associated with certain forms of arthritis, especially rheumatoid arthritis. In fact aspirin was originally invented for use in treating this disease.

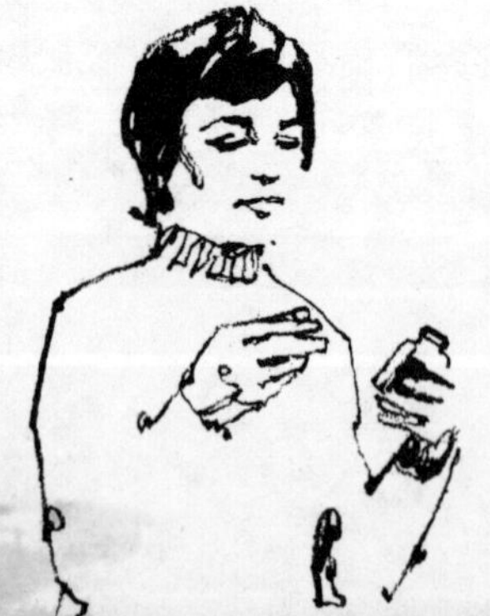

As an antiinflammatory agent aspirin helps to reduce the damage to affected joints. It also helps to reduce the swelling, stiffness, and pain caused by the inflammation. Thus, aspirin can help the arthritis patient feel better and function better.

36

One of the things your physician will have to determine is just how much aspirin you will need on a daily basis. He will also have to discover just how much aspirin your system can tolerate.

In a severe case of rheumatoid arthritis, for example, the physician will want to keep the level of aspirin intake as high as possible. And he will want this dosage continued, on a daily basis, even when the condition begins to improve, so he can maintain the antiinflammatory effect.

ASPIRIN CAN HAVE SIDE EFFECTS

As he begins treatment, the physician will soon learn how much aspirin his patient can tolerate. If the dosage is too high, the patient may report a sensation like a ringing in the ears or experience slight deafness. Aspirin overdosage may also cause headache, dizziness, dimness of vision, mental confusion, nausea, vomiting, diarrhea and gastric irritation. These symptoms will usually disappear when the dosage is reduced.

Some patients, however, will not be able to tolerate aspirin at all. It may cause an upset stomach. Or the patient may have another condition, such as peptic ulcers, which would be aggravated by taking aspirin. Some patients are also allergic to aspirin. There are varieties of aspirin which are coated to make it more tolerable.

Physicians have found that aspirin is a safe and reliable drug for the great majority of arthritic patients. It is sometimes used alone, but it can also be used in combination with other drugs when prescribed by a physician.

DRUGS FOR OSTEOARTHRITIS

No two osteoarthritic patients have exactly the same condition. For this reason there is no single drug or combination of drugs that will be used for all patients. Aspirin is the most widely used, but there are other drugs the physician may prescribe, depending on the severity of the condition.

One drug used in the treatment of osteo is phenylbutazone. This drug will not put a stop to the disease, but it may be used to treat acute outbreaks of pain for a short and limited period of time. Another medication, relatively new, which shows promise in bringing relief to osteo patients, is indomethacin. This is an antiinflammatory drug.

Not all patients can tolerate indomethacin, however; but if the side effects are not serious this drug can be beneficial in long-term treatment. It is particularly useful in relieving the pain caused by osteoarthritis of the hip. When the pain is severe, the physician may also turn to one of the more powerful pain-killing drugs.

HORMONE AND OTHER INJECTIONS

When a woman develops arthritis during the menopause, sometimes her physician will prescribe a hormone injection to bring relief to the arthritic symptoms. But hormone injections, or injections of vitamins for that matter, only bring temporary relief. They will not cure the arthritis.

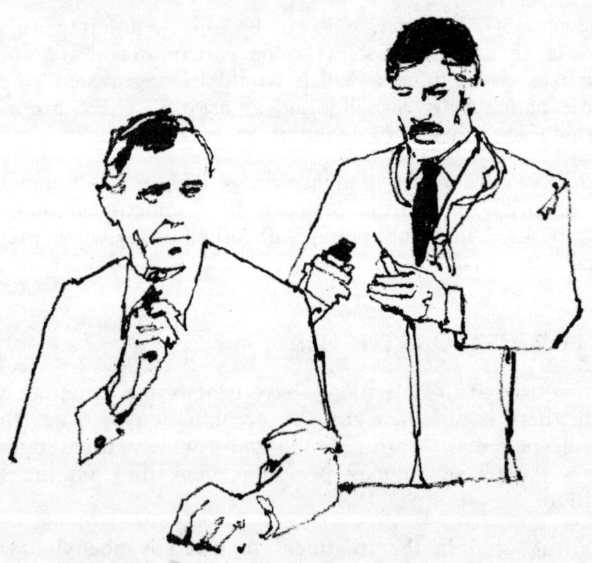

Injections of cortisone or other cortisone-derivative compounds are sometimes used to bring relief to the diseased joint when the inflammation is particularly painful. Again, this treatment will only bring temporary relief and may not have any significant effect on the progress of the disease. It will, however, reduce the inflammation in the tissues surrounding the affected joint.

MEDICATION FOR RHEUMATOID ARTHRITIS

Aspirin was originally invented for the treatment of rheumatoid arthritis. It is still considered the most important drug for use in this disease because of its ability to reduce the inflammation of the joints. Some of the other drugs already described, such as phenylbutazone and indomethacin, are also sometimes used if the patient is able to tolerate them.

When the rheumatoid arthritis attack is acute, the physician may prescribe the use of cortisone or one of its derivatives to be taken by mouth. These drugs, which are classified as "corticosteroids," are produced from a substance found in the outer layer of the adrenal glands, located just above the kidneys. They are extremely powerful in their ability to reduce the inflammation in joints. But they can also have serious side effects. For this reason the number of doses and the amount of dosage will be limited. When the cortisone treatment comes to an end, the arthritic symptoms may reappear and they may even seem worse than they were before such treatment.

SIDE EFFECTS OF CORTICOSTEROIDS

Doctors are extremely cautious in prescribing cortisone or any of the other steroids because of the side effects that can result if the patient is kept on this treatment too long. One particularly bothersome side effect is abnormal deposits of fat. "Moon face" is one of the forms this side effect takes. In other words, the patient develops a swollen, enlarged face. It is also not unusual for a patient who has taken too much cortisone to be affected mentally. This can range from insomnia to depression.

A patient can also experience an abnormal growth of hair, or his bones can become so weak that they break easily. Because this remarkable medication suddenly makes him feel well again and completely free from joint pain, the patient may throw caution to the winds. Through excessive physical activity he can aggravate the condition of his joints.

When used in excessive amounts steroids also tend to cover up the symptoms of infection. A patient can have a serious infection without knowing it. By the time it is discovered, it can be very difficult to treat, because in addition, corticosteroids at times decrease resistance to infection.

For these reasons steroid treatment is usually reserved only for severely ill patients to give temporary relief while other treatment is continued. Steroids are used only as part of a comprehensive program and never as primary treatment.

GOLD TREATMENT

Gold treatment has never been universally used by physicians in treatment of rheumatoid or other forms of arthritis, but recent studies have shown that this treatment can be very beneficial for many patients. One of the problems with gold treatment is related to the toxicity of the gold compounds used. Some patients cannot tolerate it. For this reason the doses have to be very carefully regulated, and patients will need regular complete blood counts and urinalyses during the course of treatment to guard against potentially hazardous side effects.

ANTIMALARIAL DRUGS

Another treatment that is sometimes used by physicians is the use of antimalarial drugs. These are all derivatives of quinine. When used over a long period of time antimalarial drugs have been found to reduce the symptoms of rheumatoid arthritis. These drugs may also be toxic and require expert supervision so as to prevent retinal and other ocular side effects.

DRUGS USED IN GOUT

Probably the best known drug used in the treatment of gout is colchicine. This drug is produced from the autumn crocus, which in Latin is known as colchicum. Use of this drug dates back thousands of years.

Colchicine was used alone or in combination with other drugs up to the 17th century when it suddenly (and regrettably) fell out of favor with contemporary physicians. By that time the combination of drugs used with colchicine produced a number of nauseous concoctions used as purgatives. It was not until two centuries later that colchicine was reintroduced as a medication for the treatment of gout.

This drug can have a very pronounced effect on gout, but it does not appear to have any effect on other forms of arthritis. It is for this reason that physicians often use colchicine to diagnose a gout condition. If the treatment with colchicine is effective, the patient has gout and not another form of arthritis.

For many years colchicine has been the drug of choice in controlling acute attacks of gout because of its ability to reduce inflammation. But it is a powerful drug and can sometimes produce uncomfortable side effects, such as abdominal cramps and diarrhea. Presently other drugs, such as phenylbutazone, are preferred by many rheumatologists in treating acute attacks of gout.

If used in time colchicine almost always prevents the acute gouty attack. But it has to be taken long before the attack reaches its peak. When used in this way, only small amounts of the drug (such as one or two tablets a day) will be necessary to contain the attack. This reduces the possibility of undesirable side effects very significantly. Sometimes colchicine is given intravenously, and this can result in remarkably fast relief of joint pain and swelling. The patient's condition can then be managed through oral dosage.

PROBENECID AND SULFINPYRAZONE

Two of the most effective drugs in bringing relief to the gout sufferer are probenecid and sulfinpyrazone. Probenecid has been used for a number of years to prevent the accumulation of uric acid in the body. It accomplishes this by increasing the amount of excretion of uric acid by the kidney. Probenecid will not reduce the pain associated with gout, but through continued use it can help prevent an acute attack.

Sulfinpyrazone is a newer uricosuric agent which also prevents the accumulation of uric acid. It is often used alone but sometimes in combination with probenecid. Doctors have found it particularly useful in patients who are unresponsive to probenecid or who can't tolerate it.

ALLOPURINOL

Allopurinol is one of the newest drugs used in the treatment of gout. Its discovery was hailed as one of the most important breakthroughs in the treatment of this disease. Whereas probenecid helps the body get rid of the excess uric acid, allopurinol acts to inhibit the body's *production* of uric acid. This is accomplished by limiting the action of the enzyme, xanthine oxidase, which is directly involved in the production of uric acid.

Minor and infrequent side effects have been associated with the use of allopurinol. These include abdominal cramps and a mild fever; but they usually occur only when the patient first begins to use the drug. Most patients are able to tolerate allopurinol with no discomfort. Very rarely, it can cause serious complications.

This drug has also been found to be particularly useful in preventing the formation of kidney stones because of its ability to reduce the flow of uric acid through the kidneys. This makes it particularly useful for treatment of patients who would otherwise tend to form kidney stones.

CHAPTER 8

When Surgery Is Used To Bring Relief

REMARKABLE ADVANCES IN SURGERY to bring relief and a new lease on life to patients crippled by arthritis were dramatically described by science writer Arthur J. Snider when he wrote:

"At a recent wedding reception, the belle of the ball was not the bride but a 44-year-old housewife who danced all night. There's nothing new about doing the hokey-pokey, mamba or samba at a wedding except that the last time most of the astonished guests had seen her, this woman was grotesquely crippled from a 30-year siege of rheumatoid arthritis. She slithered along with a shuffle-waddle-wobble gait, knock-knees locked and bent like a skier, toes turned in. With hips frozen in a fixed position, her mobile power came from twisting them from one side and then the other."

Mr. Snider went on to report that the formerly crippled arthritis victim could now walk normally as the result of an operation in which she received two artificial hip joints and the first of two artificial knee joints. She was also scheduled for an operation to receive new artificial joints of plastic to repair her gnarled and stiffened fingers so she could open and close her hand. The joints in her other hand had previously been fused to relieve the pain before the plastic joints became available. As Mr. Snider expressed it, "The operating room is a growing new frontier for arthritic relief."

WHEN SURGERY IS RECOMMENDED

Severe crippling from osteoarthritis or rheumatoid arthritis is not uncommon, particularly in patients who have not received the benefits of early and continued treatment by a physician. Any arthritic condition can lead to crippling if the disease is allowed to run its course unchecked.

The result is always predictable: continued inflammation of the synovial membrane permits corrosive enzymes to attack the remaining healthy cells. This causes destruction in the soft tissue surrounding a joint as well as in the cartilage and bone. If the destruction is great enough the sufferer's bones will become scarred and pitted and will produce excruciating pain during movement. When this condition develops in a patient's hip, it can severely restrict his ability to walk.

Specialists in hip surgery at the Mayo Clinic, where more than 2,000 total hip replacements were performed in a two-and-a-half year period, recently reported on their increasing success with this operation. They also discussed the number of considerations they make before surgery is recommended.

"We must analyze the amount of pain," stated Mark B. Coventry, M.D., "and whether it is tolerable or not; whether the patient can carry on with his or her job; whether, even though one can work, there has been any loss in ability to do avocational activities and keep happy; whether the patient can rest comfortably at night; and, very importantly, whether we can demonstrate by the natural history of the disease and with serial roentgenograms and examinations that the arthritis is progressing and will ultimately become much worse."

Total hip replacement is a dramatic example of a new era in orthopedic surgery designed to alleviate the severe crippling of arthritis. Operations are now also being performed to replace badly crippled knee joints with artificial devices as well as joints in the fingers and wrists.

In total hip replacement a ball and socket device made of metal and plastic is inserted in place of the badly damaged joint. This can restore normal mobility almost completely. Thousands of these operations are now performed each year. Many other surgical procedures are now being developed by those involved in a new field called "bioengineering" in which physicians, engineers and other specialists are combining their efforts to develop artificial devices to replace badly damaged joints in the human body.

NEW MATERIALS BODY WILL TOLERATE

This already has led to the development of new materials which the body will tolerate, such as vitalium. This is an alloy composed of

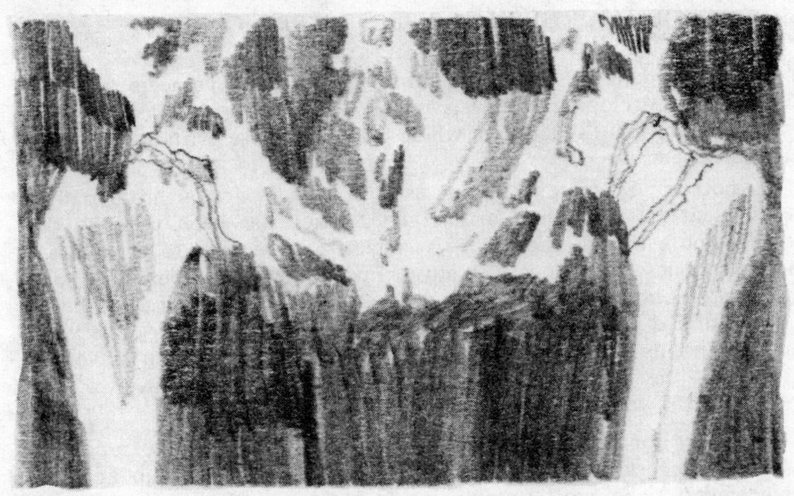

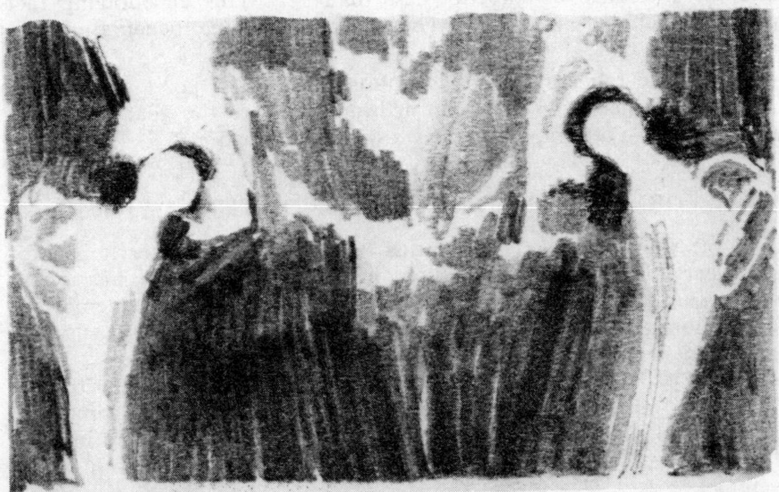

Drawing at top shows deterioration of hip joints due to arthritis. The drawing below shows hip joints that have been replaced by artificial devices.

cobalt, chromium, and molybdenum. Today's bioengineers are concerned with developing materials which will not be corroded by secretions in the patient's body or which will not cause irritation or other harmful effects.

Another new material being used in surgery for arthritic patients is a cement called methyl methacrylate, which has been used by dentists for more than a decade. This cement can be used to form a synthetic bone base to connect the hip or knee bones of patients with metal and plastic joints. Before this cement became available, surgeons had to screw artificial joints into the adjoining bone. In time these joints would loosen, bringing a return of the patient's pain and difficulty in movement. At present the use of methyl methacrylate has been limited to older patients, with very few exceptions.

Surgery for the arthritic patient is at best a complex procedure. As in all surgery there are risks involved, particularly in hip and knee replacements. The most notable is the incidence of infection. Yet, in its report on the first 333 hip replacement operations, the Mayo Clinic found the incidence of infection less than 1%. This encouraging fact should be included in Dr. Coventry's listing of the benefits of this operation.

"Complete relief of pain, restoration of stability, good motion—all of which are usual after total hip arthroplasty—are the goal," declared Dr. Coventry. "Total hip surgery is a dynamic situation."

OTHER FORMS OF SURGERY FOR ARTHRITIS

Surgery for the relief of arthritis sufferers has been performed for many years, though the procedures have been limited to more conservative surgery. This includes the removal of the synovial membrane. This membrane is the center of the inflammation which causes ultimate damage to the bone, cartilage and other connective tissues. When medication fails to bring improvement and when further deterioration of the joint appears inevitable, this surgical procedure is sometimes recommended. Removal of the synovial membrane, if performed in time, will help prevent the severe erosion of bone and cartilage which causes crippling.

Another common operation for arthritis is the replacement of seriously damaged finger joints with flexible silicone rubber implants. Before the artificial finger joints are implanted they have usually been

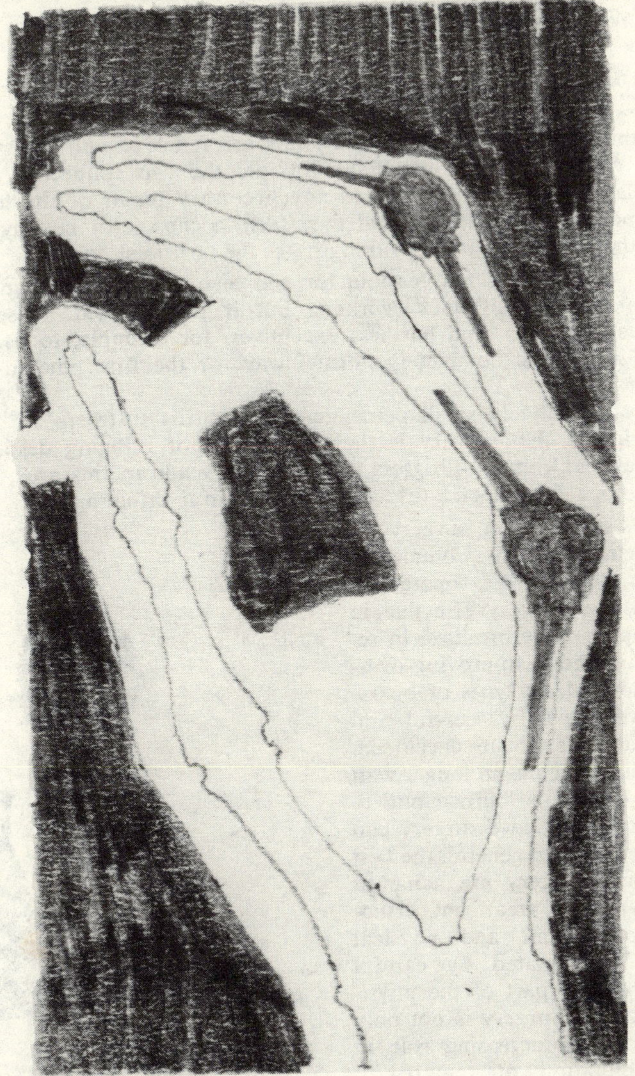

The shaded areas in the fingers indicate where artificial joints have been placed to restore movability.

bent by test machines for 90 million times or more without breaking to insure their stability.

In this operation the deformed joints are removed and the surgeon makes a channel for the artificial joint into the two connecting bones. The implant is then positioned and any necessary repair of the tendons is then made. As the fingers heal they form a capsule of healthy tissue around the implants, adding strength to the artificial joints.

This operation is not feasible for people in strenuous occupations, such as laborers and dock workers, but it has enabled housewives, secretaries, salesmen, and business executives, for example, to use their hands in an almost completely normal way for the first time in many years.

Only a relatively small percentage of arthritis sufferers are so severely crippled that surgery is the only means of bringing desperately needed relief. Dramatic progress is now being made in this area, bringing new hope for an end to serious and painful crippling.

In its statement on surgery for arthritis, the Arthritis Foundation declared, "Orthopedic operations on joints can be very effective in preventing some deformities, in relieving pain and in improving overall function. Many types of operations have proved successful and new operations are being developed. Orthopedic surgeons no longer wait until the disease is 'burned out' to operate if they believe surgery can help the patient. In general, the best results from surgery are achieved when the medical treatment, orthopedic management and physical care are coordinated by careful planning on the part of the physicians involved. Surgery is not only playing an ever-increasing role in the rehabilitation of the handicapped patient, but now is useful in preventing deformities."

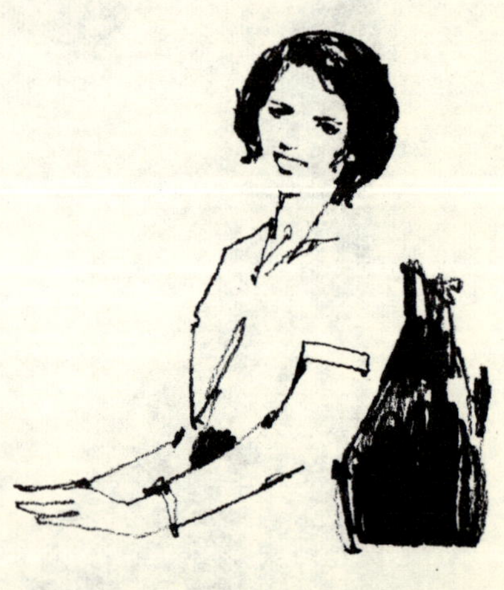

Surgery can be useful in preventing deformities.

CHAPTER 9

Physical Therapy, Exercise and Rest

IF YOUR ARTHRITIC CONDITION is severe enough, your doctor may recommend that you consult with a physiatrist, a physician who specializes in physical medicine. He will develop a program of exercises for you to help prevent crippling. The physiatrist, in turn, may suggest that your exercise program be started under the supervision of a person trained in this area such as a physical therapist, an occupational therapist or a public health nurse.

The reason you may need supervision in getting started is that without proper instruction you may unintentionally do damage to your affected joints. A physical therapist, for example, will demonstrate the proper methods to be used in performing stretching exercises. This is within her area of special training, and before she introduces the exercises to you she will have consulted with your personal physician or physiatrist.

If your doctor arranges for you to see an occupational therapist, this specialist will show you how you can organize your work and other daily activities so you can perform them without unnecessary difficulty. The occupational therapist can also introduce you to self-help devices that will make your daily activities more comfortable by helping you to avoid undue strain on painful joints.

FINDING THE PROPER BALANCE
BETWEEN REST AND EXERCISE

Your physician will assist you in developing the proper balance between rest and exercise. Both are extremely important in the management of your arthritic condition. If you get too much rest this can increase the pain and stiffness in muscles and joints. If you get too much exercise, on the other hand, there is the danger that you will increase the damage to your joints as well as the level of pain. The severity of your condition will be the guiding factor.

Generally speaking, if your joints are inflamed, if you have a fever and feel fatigued, your body needs as much rest as possible. If these conditions exist they indicate that your entire system is affected. Rest will help to reduce the inflammation and its consequent effects on your joints and other parts of your body.

There are many ways you can rest in order to make this experience as beneficial as possible. For example, always try to keep a correct posture so you won't be giving undue strain to any of your joints. Avoid standing for long periods of time. Sit down whenever possible since this will bring rest to your weight-bearing joints such as the hips, knees, ankles, and feet. If you feel the need to lie down during the day, keep in mind that it is better to take several short periods of rest rather than one long period.

EXERCISES YOUR PHYSICIAN MAY PRESCRIBE

There are four types of exercises that physicians may prescribe for arthritic patients: range of motion exercises, strengthening exercises, stretching exercises, and functional exercises.

Every joint in your body has a "range of motion," in other words it can be moved to certain limits in various directions. When your doctor recommends that you perform *range of motion exercises* for specific joints he will ask you to move them in all possible directions for a certain period of time each day. This will help restore normal movement.

Strengthening exercises are used to increase the power or "work-ability" of muscles. An example of this is the "muscle setting" exercise, sometimes referred to as an isometric or muscle-tightening exercise. This will aid painful joints by strengthening them with a minimum of actual joint motion.

When your joints are so stiff that you can't move them within a normal range, your doctor may prescribe a *stretching exercise*. Usually this kind of exercise will be done under the direct supervision of your physician or a physical therapist.

Functional exercises are used to improve the patient's ability to perform some of the daily tasks necessary in caring for himself, such as tying shoes, buttoning shirts or blouses, zipping up skirts or trousers. These are basically arm and finger exercises to help the arthritic patient take care of his personal needs.

ARM AND HAND EXERCISES

In its booklet, "Home Care Programs in Arthritis," the Arthritis Foundation describes a number of exercises that physicians may prescribe to their patients in order to improve their abilities to use their hands, arms, and legs as well as to improve their posture.

Arm Exercise. Standing as erect as possible, raise your arms as high over your head as you can. Be sure to keep your elbows straight. Now swing your arms out and down to your sides. Then rotate your arms in as large a circle as possible.

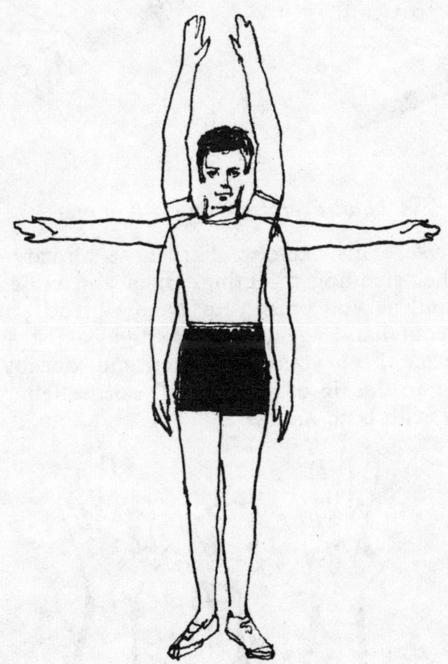

Illustration of arm exercise.

Hand Exercise. Take a hammer and grab the handle near the hammer's head. Now, keeping your upper arm by your side, bend your elbow to a right angle. Then turn your wrist from left to right repeatedly, letting the weight of the hammer turn your hand over as far as possible in each motion. Perform this exercise with both hands several times. Once this exercise becomes less strenuous you can shift your grip further down toward the other end of the handle so the weight of the hammer is more noticeable.

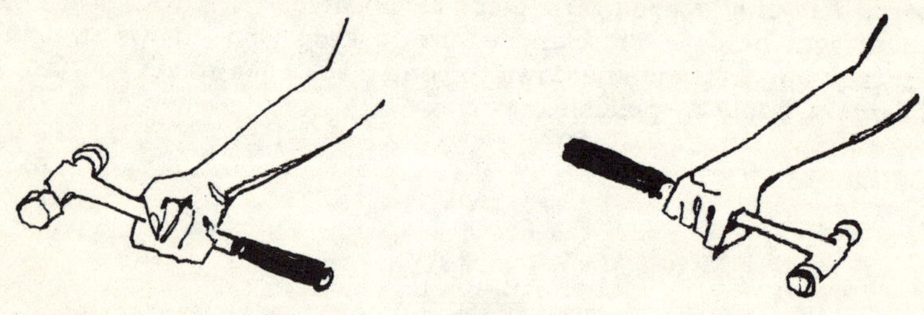

A hand exercise using a hammer.

Finger Exercise. This exercise, like those already mentioned, can be performed either standing or sitting. Open and close your hand in a regular rhythm, and as you open your hand, spread your fingers wide. When you close your hand again, make as tight a fist as you can. Now for a change of pace, keep your hand open and, one by one, touch the end of each finger to the tip of your thumb so the letter "O" is formed. Do these exercises with both hands.

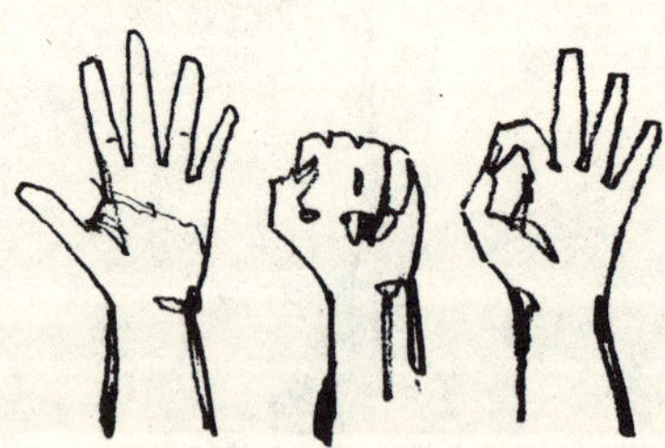

Finger exercises.

Leg Exercise. One leg exercise your physician may recommend involves bending the knees. First, lie on your back and then bend your right knee up toward your chest. When doing this your knee and hip should be bent as far as possible. You may want to use your hands to pull your knee up toward you. Hold this position for a few seconds and then slowly lower your leg, making sure your knee is kept straight. Repeat these movements several times, using both legs.

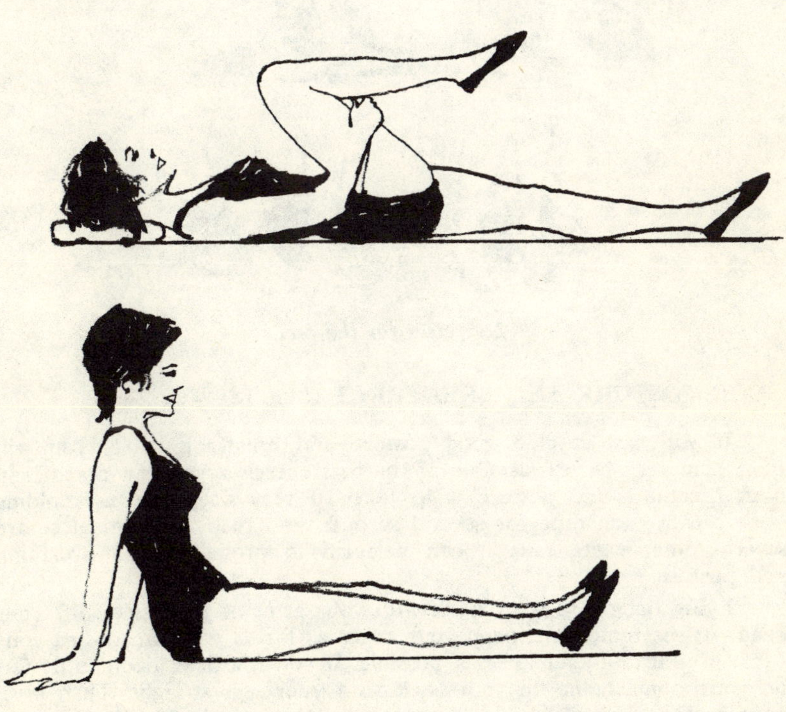

Leg exercise involving the bending of the knees.

Exercises for the Feet. Take your shoes off and sit in a chair with your feet flat on the floor. Raise your toes as high as you can, while keeping your heels flat against the floor. Now reverse this procedure. Keep your toes flat against the floor and raise your heels as high as you can. Here's another variation: with your feet flat on the floor, lift the inside of each foot and roll the weight over on the outside of the foot. If possible, keep your toes curled down.

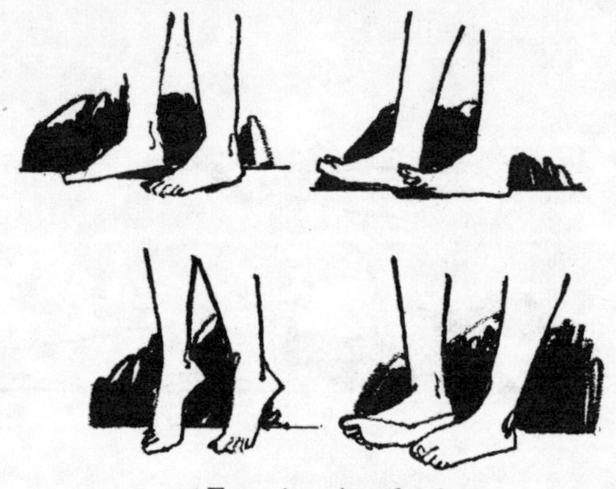

Exercises for the feet.

GOOD POSTURE AND BREATHING HABITS

If you can develop good posture and breathing habits you will find them very beneficial. One of the best exercises you can do to help both breathing and posture is to take 10 very deep breaths, holding your breath each time for several seconds and then relaxing. Here are several other exercises you can perform to promote good breathing and posture:

Lying flat on your stomach with your arms at your sides, lift your head. At the same time, bend your knees as far as you can toward your back, even lifting your knees if possible. If you find it difficult to lie flat on your stomach, lie on your back with your legs straight. Then push your heels and shoulders down against the floor (or bed) and raise your buttocks. Hold this position for several seconds.

Another exercise you can perform while flat on your back is to put your hands on your chest and breathe in deeply. At the same time push your ribs against your hands. Hold for a few seconds and then breathe out.

APPLYING HEAT AND COLD

To give temporary relief when the discomfort from the aches and pains of arthritis are particularly severe, your physician may recommend hot or cold applications. A cold compress such as an ice bag will produce a numbing effect and thereby give some relief from pain. Applications of heat will tend to relax tense muscles and can be particularly beneficial before you begin any exercise. There are a number of devices you can use to produce the desired heat, among them, heat lamps, heating pads, paraffin baths, warm compresses, and warm baths.

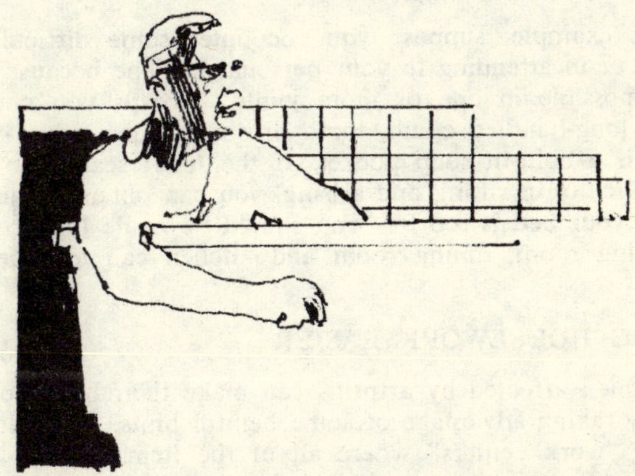

A warm bath is an effective way to apply heat to several joints at the same time.

One of the most effective ways to apply heat to several joints at the same time is to take a warm bath. The water should not be too hot. It is usually recommended that you not spend more than 20 minutes in the tub. Staying in a warm bath for longer than 20 minutes may make you feel tired and weak.

Keep in mind that any method of applying heat or cold to affected arthritic joints should be done only under a doctor's direction.

CHAPTER 10

Self-Help Devices

IF YOU ARE LIKE MOST ARTHRITIC PATIENTS, the last thing you want to do is think of yourself as an invalid. You want to be as independent as possible in taking care of your personal needs and in performing any of the functions related to work or recreation. In spite of the pride you may take in being as independent as possible, however, you may be able to benefit from some of the many self-help devices available to arthritis sufferers.

For example, suppose you encounter some difficulty in dressing yourself or in attending to your personal hygiene because of the limited motion possible in one or more joints. Perhaps you could benefit by using a long-handled comb, tooth brush, or shoe horn, or a washcloth mitt with a built-in soap pocket. If the toilet seat is so low that you have difficulty in sitting and arising, you can obtain a raised toilet seat. Perhaps your bed is too low and should be made higher. The chairs in your living room, dining room and kitchen can also be raised.

MAKING HOUSEWORK EASIER

Women affected by arthritis can make their household tasks much easier by taking advantage of some helpful hints. For instance, you can organize "work centers" where all of the items needed for a specific job are kept within easy reach. This is important in avoiding unnecessary strain and fatigue.

When ironing, for example, have your moistened clothes, as well as a rack on which to hang the ironed clothes, within easy reaching distance. This will make it possible for you to reach the clothes, iron them, and hang them up while in a seated position.

When preparing a meal, organize this activity so you can move

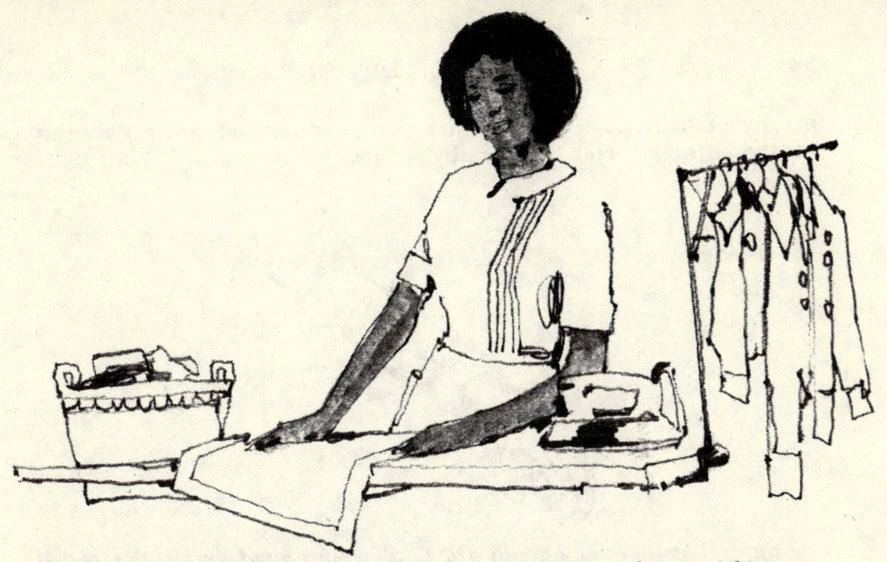

from the refrigerator to the counter top, sink and stove without taking a lot of unnecessary steps. This is particularly important to the arthritic patient with weak legs or feet.

To relieve the strain on weakened arms and hands, use electric jar and can openers. Keep your food in lightweight plastic or aluminum foil containers.

For ease in moving things about, consider using a tea cart or small table with casters. This can be used for transporting laundry, dishes, and food as well as cleaning supplies.

USE OF SPLINTS

When splints are recommended for an arthritic condition they are usually made from a lightweight plastic. Your physician will also make certain that the splint is fitted very carefully to the affected joint. A splint may be recommended for one of several reasons. Your joint may be inflamed and the splint will help rest it and prevent or correct any potential deformity. Or it may be that he wants to be sure the joint is protected from unnecessary stress. Splints for arthritic patients are usually partially open splints which permit movement, when necessary, of the affected joints or nearby joints.

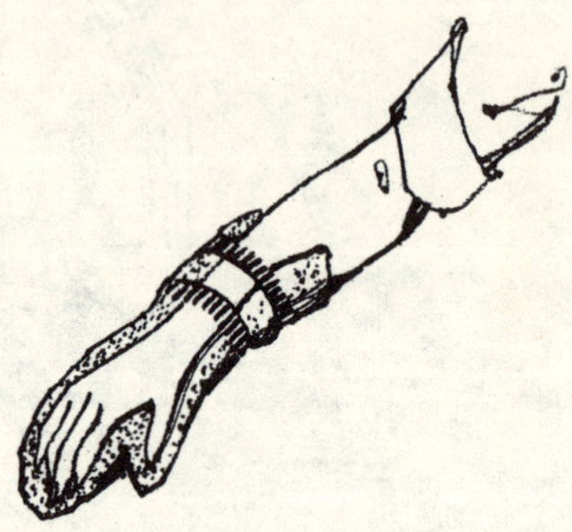

Resting splints like the one illustrated above are used during rest periods and when the patient is sleeping.

If a joint is acutely inflamed, your physician may advise you to wear a splint throughout the day and night. As your condition improves, he may ask you to leave the splint on for only part of the day. Sometimes it may be necessary to have a new splint made so the soft tissues in the joint can be stretched to a better position.

Physicians have found splints particularly helpful in treating arthritic hands, wrists, and knees. A *resting* splint for the hand and wrist is used during rest periods and when the patient is sleeping. This will help prevent deformities and, at the same time, is no deterrent to exercise. In fact, your physician may feel that it is particularly important that you perform certain prescribed exercises to help prevent any crippling or deforming effects of an arthritis attack. Exercises to help set the muscles and keep them functioning can be performed even though you may be wearing a hand and wrist splint.

Another type of splint is the functional wrist splint. While the patient is wearing this splint his inflamed wrist is rested and supported but he can still move his fingers for whatever functions that are necessary. To give rest to the knee, there is the "long leg splint." This is also used to prevent the knee from becoming stiff in a bent position. The long leg splint is also helpful when the patient is standing or walking because of the protection it gives to the knee joint.

HELP FOR ARTHRITIC FEET

If your feet are affected by arthritis, your physician may advise you to wear certain kinds of shoes in order to prevent any unnecessary deformity. They will also help you to maintain a correct posture.

Both men and women patients with arthritic feet are usually advised to wear Oxford shoes with a "straight" last and heels that are low and wide. If he feels that you need help in preventing your feet from rolling inward, your physician will recommend that you get shoes with a long counter or Thomas heel. To relieve pressure on the ball of the foot, he may recommend that you get shoes with a metatarsal bar.

In some patients with arthritic feet there is a tendency toward an inward turning of the feet. To prevent this your physician may suggest that you get shoes with wedges. If your feet are badly deformed and painful, it may be necessary for you to get shoes that are specially molded to give you the relief you need in walking.

CANES AND CRUTCHES TO PREVENT CRIPPLING

Many arthritic patients who have a certain amount of mobility but could benefit from a self-help device such as a cane or crutches oftentimes resist the suggestion. After all, they say, I'm not a cripple, not yet! The physician has to explain to them that their arthritic joints, in particular the weight-bearing joints such as the hips, knees, ankles and feet, may be damaged if they are sufficiently inflamed by arthritis. By using a cane or crutches the patient takes much of the stress and strain off the inflamed joints and helps prevent unnecessary deformity. If the inflammation is very acute, of course, the patient will be confined to his bed.

Two types of cane that are commonly used are the "C" cane and the "T" cane. Your physician will prescribe the type best fitted to your condition. Oftentimes arthritic patients find the "T" cane easier to hold onto. The standard length for canes is 36", but if you are shorter or taller than average it will be necessary to use canes that have been fitted to your height. It is also important that they be rubber-tipped to prevent slipping.

The proper procedure for using a cane is to hold it in the hand that is opposite to the arthritic hip, knee, ankle or foot. Move the cane at the same time you move the leg affected by arthritis.

Crutches have to be measured to the patient. Those used by arthritis patients are usually of the underarm type with a shoulder piece and handgrip of rubber or soft plastic. The rubber tip on the bottom should be at least 1½ " high. In using crutches it is important to keep in mind that when you are standing still you should be resting your weight. When walking with crutches you should be carrying your weight on the hand grips and not on the shoulder pieces.

TIPS ON USE OF A WHEELCHAIR

The arthritic patient who has to use a wheelchair either all or part of the time, whether it be at work or at home, has to learn the "rules of the roll." At home, for example, the patient should use the wheelchair in rooms and halls that are large or wide enough to permit him to turn around with ease. If door thresholds are unusually high they should be removed or replaced with lower thresholds.

Doors that slide or fold are much more practical for the wheelchair patient than doors with hinges because they are much easier to open or close.

If it is difficult to use a work counter or other work surfaces, a wheelchair tray may serve as well. Otherwise it will be necessary to provide for leg space under counters.

The physician will advise the wheelchair patient in the selection of the most practical wheelchair for his needs. Among the usual recommendations is that it be light in weight with a firm, flat seat. It should also provide the proper support for the patient's back and legs, allowing an adequate degree of bend for hips and knees.

For the patient with arthritis of the knees the wheelchair should have leg extensions which will permit the knees to be kept straight. For all arthritic patients the wheelchair should have removable arms to make it easier for the patient to transfer to and from the toilet, bed, or chair.

WHERE TO FIND SELF-HELP DEVICES

The following firms have been recommended by the Arthritis Foundation as reliable sources for self-help devices:

BE OK SALES CO.

Box 32, Brookfield, Ill. 60513. Self-help aids, including built-up eating utensils, Velcro tape closure, personal hygiene aids, kitchen aids, shoe fasteners and stocking aids.

CLEO LIVING AIDS

3957 Mayfield Rd., Cleveland, Ohio 44121. Self-help equipment including clothing, eating aids, shower and bath devices. Catalogue.

FASHIONABLE, INC.

Mrs. Van Davis Odell, P.O. Box 23188, Fort Lauderdale, Fla., 33307. Mail order clothes for the handicapped woman, featuring specially designed undergarments. Catalogue.

G. E. MILLER, INC.

484 South Broadway, Yonkers, N.Y. 10705. Physical medicine and self-help equipment, including stocking and dressing aids, eating utensils, homemaking equipment.

REHAB AIDS

5931 S.W. 8th Street, Box 612, Miami, Fla. 33144. Mail order firm specializing in self-help devices. Catalogue.

SHELTERED WORKSHOP FOR THE DISABLED, INC.

200 Court Street, Binghampton, N.Y. 13902. Manufacture "U-shaped" stocking aid. Pamphlets.

VOCATIONAL GUIDANCE & REHABILITATION SERVICES

2289 East 55th Street, Cleveland, Ohio 44103. Clothing for handicapped women, including dresses, suits, slips, separates, and accessories. A few items for men. Pamphlet.

WINCO PRODUCTS

Winfield Co., Inc., 3062 46th Avenue, N., St. Petersburg, Fla. 33714. Self-help equipment including raised toilet seats, shower/commode chairs, walkers, safety bars.

CHAPTER 11

The Importance of Diet

"The healthiest people are those who pay attention to themselves, what they do, and what they eat. I tend to think that the French proverb, 'Death enters by the mouth,' is picturesque but a little exaggerated; we do not really dig our graves with our teeth. Still, we all should eat a properly balanced diet, one adequate in calories, with a maximum of protein, enough vitamins and minerals, and a minimum of fat and starches."

This is the advice offered by rheumatologist John J. Calabro, M.D., and it is good advice that doctors frequently and repeatedly give to their arthritic patients. For sufferers from osteo or rheumatoid arthritis there is no specific "arthritic diet," designed to bring relief to their condition. Diet, however, is particularly important to your overall condition.

If your physician should discover a deficiency in your diet, he will recommend certain foods to bring your nutritional intake up to par. But, generally speaking, there is no known diet or specific food that will help cure your arthritis. The important thing about food is the nutrition it produces, and good nutrition means eating a variety of foods that your body needs.

If an arthritic patient is overweight, the physician may recommend that the patient go on a weight-reducing diet in order to take unnecessary strain off the weight-bearing joints. As people grow older, they should eat less. According to authorities on nutrition, a simple rule of thumb to follow is: "Every 10 years eat 10 per cent less."

For the underweight arthritic patient—and this is often the case in rheumatoid arthritis patients who suffer from loss of appetite—the physician will recommend a diet that will help the patient to regain his normal weight.

Good nourishment will provide the nutritional help your arthritic joints and muscles need in order to get the greatest benefit from medication and other treatment your physician may prescribe.

FOOD AND BEVERAGE RESTRICTIONS FOR GOUT SUFFERERS

Gout patients are usually advised by their physicians to keep their weight as close as possible to normal. In some cases they may also advise that certain foods high in purine content be avoided. This will include such foods as anchovies, sardines, sweetbreads, kidney, liver, brains, meat extract (e.g. bouillon), and gravies. It may also include beverages such as beer and other malt products.

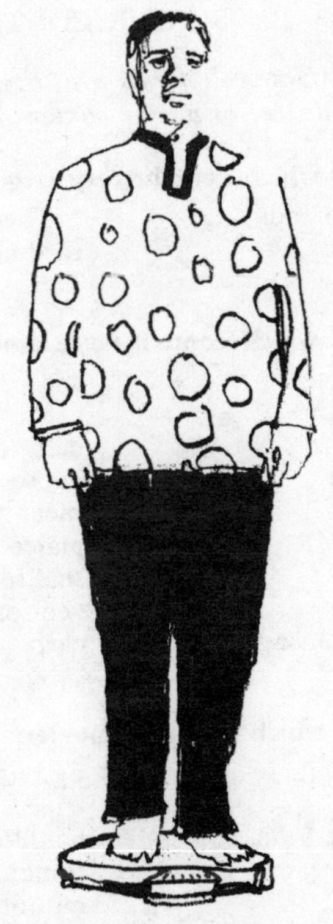

Diet, in itself, will not control the patient's gout condition. It may help to alleviate it, but it cannot prevent the occurrence of an acute attack of gout. Physicians have also found that many patients do not follow their dietary advice as regularly as they should. Fortunately, the medication now used for gout can do a great deal to prevent the overproduction of uric acid and help the body get rid of the uric acid it produces.

The following listing of the purine content of certain foods is given here as an aid to the gout sufferer in selecting the foods that will be most beneficial and in avoiding those foods which may aggravate his condition.

PURINE CONTENT OF CERTAIN FOODS

(Note: all foods are listed from high to low, according to the degree of purine content.)

Foods which contain very large amounts of purine bodies:

sweetbreads	gravies	meat extracts
brains	sardines in oil	liver (calf & beef)
anchovies	kidney (beef)	

Foods which contain large amounts of purine bodies:

bacon	sheep	halibut
codfish	veal	partridge
perch	calf tongue	pork
pigeon	goose	squab
rabbit	meat soups	chicken soup
turkey	plaice	lentils
beef	shellfish	pheasant
duck	venison	quail
liver sausage	carp	trout
pike		

Foods which contain a moderate amount of purine bodies:

asparagus	oysters	ham
crab	tripe	mushrooms
kidney beans	bouillon	salmon
navy beans	finnan haddie	whitefish
spinach	mutton	chicken
bluefish	peas	herring
eel	tuna fish	oatmeal
lima beans	cauliflower	shad

Also whole grain bread and breadstuff:

graham bread	rye krisp	whole grain bread
rye bread	graham crackers	

Also whole grain cereals:

bran	puffed wheat	shredded wheat
rolled wheat	cracked wheat	graham porridge
bran flakes	malt breakfast food	wheat flakes

Foods which contain an insignificant amount of purine or no purine:

Beverages:
carbonated, chocolate, coffee, cocoa, tea, fruit juices
Butter*
Breads and breadstuffs:
butter thins, rusk, corn bread, soda crackers, corn sticks, water rolls, french bread, white bread, gluten bread, zwieback
Caviar
Cereal:
grits, white cornmeal, puffed rice, rice krispies, rice flakes, corn flakes, refined wheat cereal
Miscellaneous cereal products:
arrowroot, spaghetti, hominy, tapioca, macaroni, vermicelli, noodles, sago
Cheese of all kinds*
Eggs
Fats of all kinds (but eat in moderation)*
Fruits of all kinds
Gelatin
Milk
buttermilk, condensed milk, malted milk
Nuts of all kinds*
peanut butter*
Pies (except mincemeat)
Shad roe
Sugar and sweets
Vegetables:
artichokes, cucumber, rutabagas, broccoli, celery, endive, lettuce, turnips, string beans, sauerkraut, corn, brussel sprouts, carrots, pumpkin, okra, beet greens, kohlrabi, beets, summer squash, tomato, cabbage, parsnips, eggplant, dandelion greens, potato (white & sweet)
Vegetable and cream soups (to be made with allowed vegetables & without meat stock)
Vitamin concentrates
Codliver oil, halibut oil, yeast

*These foods are high in fat.

CHAPTER 12

Beware
of Fraudulent
Claims

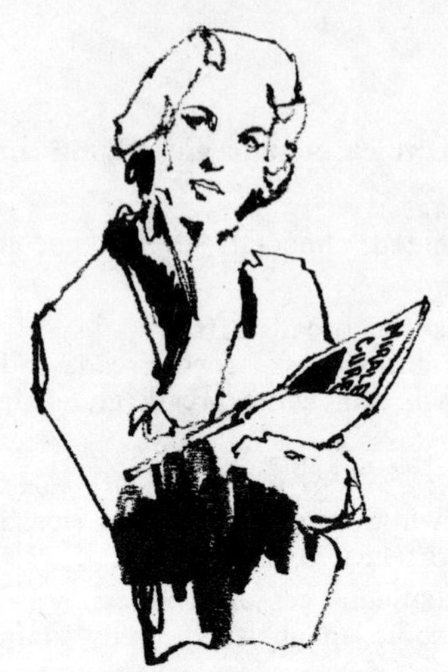

ACUPUNCTURE AND "MOON DUST" are two of the newest lures for gullible arthritis patients who are being bilked out of thousands of dollars. They both represent a despicable practice that has been going on for decades in this country.

The publicity given to the use of acupuncture in Red China as an anesthetic in surgery and dentistry and the moon landings of the astronauts have triggered these latest developments in arthritis frauds.

These lures have joined a long list of phoney cure-alls tied directly to developments in science and medicine. When electricity was discovered, for example, arthritis charlatans touted electrical devices to bring an end to arthritis suffering. With the discovery of radio, there was "radionics." When the atom bomb was invented, based on a chain reaction from uranium, this element was touted as a cure-all. In fact, this "cure" is still being advertised. Many, lured by false hope, are still lining up to sit in a uranium mine for $10 an hour to benefit from the "magic radiation."

Why are arthritis sufferers so eager to try any touted "cure" for their aches and pains? One reason may be that, as yet, there is no known cause and no known cure. Another reason lies in the nature of the disease itself. The arthritis sufferer may be experiencing intense pain, and then suddenly the pain begins to lessen and go away. They may be without pain for several weeks or months or even years before they suffer another attack. This sudden lessening of pain may occur when they have been tricked into taking some phoney cure. So they think that this has cured them, even though medical evidence will prove that it has not. They simply *want* to believe that they have been cured.

But, unaided by the advice of a physician (who has probably not been consulted), they walk blissfully on with complete faith in the "cure" until pains of arthritis return. They are frequently unaware of the great dangers implicit in many phoney cure-alls. Here are two examples.

Thousands of Americans have made a pilgrimage to Canada to purchase a drug called "liefcort" which is sold as a treatment for the symptoms of arthritis. The inventor of the drug's "secret formula" is a doctor named Robert E. Liefmann, who concocted the preparation in the basement of his home. Soon afterwards he began claiming miraculous success with the drug and even published an article which stated that hundreds of persons using his remedy "have now left their wheelchairs and are living normal lives and thousands of persons will soon be helped." His claims spread like wildfire throughout the North American continent and "liefcort" became Liefmann's "gold mine," at $10 for a half-ounce bottle.

WARNINGS ISSUED

The American Medical Association, the U.S. Food and Drug Administration, and the Arthritis Foundation conducted studies which proved that liefcort is a dangerous drug which contains three potent hormones: prednisone, testosterone, and estradiol. They issued warnings in an attempt to stop the fraud in its tracks.

Prednisone is sometimes used in the treatment of arthritis. But, as the AMA pointed out in its warning, prednisone is a corticosteroid and can have serious side effects if not used under a doctor's direction. These side effects can include hemorrhaging, peptic ulcers, the spontaneous fracture of bones, and mental derangement. The arthritis sufferers who came to Liefmann for his drug did not stay on for long-term treatment so he could check their reactions to the drug. They paid for the little bottle with the brown liquid and returned home.

As for testosterone and estradiol, the Food and Drug Administration pointed out that they have never been observed to exert any beneficial effect in arthritis but may produce serious side effects, such as changes in masculine and feminine characteristics. FDA analysis showed, moreover, that liefcort contained 10 times the amount of estradiol than was generally used in medication.

According to published reports on reactions to the drug, it has caused several deaths. Some women who used the drug grew beards, and some men developed breasts. One six-year-old New Jersey girl who was given the drug developed a bosom and began menstruating. She also required an operation to correct the degeneration in both hips apparently caused by the prednisone.

BANNED AS DANGEROUS

Liefcort, understandably, has been banned in the United States and declared "imminently dangerous." It is also illegal in Canada, but the law there, as in the United States, permits a licensed doctor to administer drugs to his patients in his office. Canadian officials have also suspended Liefmann's license because he has allowed unlicensed assistants to give his "treatment." They have also charged him with selling hormones without proper labels, preparing drugs under unsuitable conditions and other violations. At this writing lawsuits are still pending in Canadian courts. Liefmann is continuing his operation in Canada, however, and has since opened a "clinic" in Mexico. Meanwhile thousands of arthritis sufferers continue to risk the dangerous side effects by taking this condemned drug.

The same shenanigans are going on south of the U.S. border in Mexico. A few years ago stories came from Mexico about a miraculous new drug for arthritis developed by a Mexican physician in a town located near the Texas border.

As Lester David described it in an article published in *Good Housekeeping* magazine, "News spread and soon thousands of sufferers, hopes high, began streaming into the city. In Monroe, Louisiana, a local airlines arranged special flights to handle swarms of pain-racked arthritics. They packed the doctor's office and bought ampules of a drug which they were told would not be available in the U.S. for two years. Returning home, they asked their doctors to inject the medication, and a few did."

A number of patients made enthusiastic claims of "dramatic" relief.

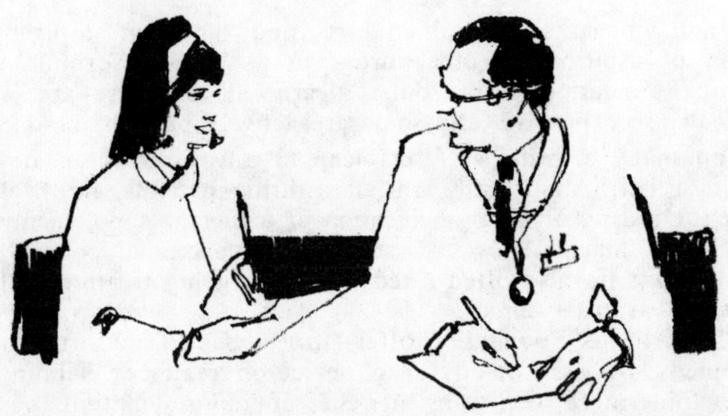

If you are tempted to try a misleadingly advertised product that promises complete relief or "cure" for your arthritis, discuss it with your physician first.

A group of arthritic patients in Louisiana even asked their congressmen to get state approval for the drug so they wouldn't have to make the trip to Mexico. This prompted an investigation, and with the help of the Food and Drug Administration the drug and its manufacturer were identified. When the report was made public, the "miraculous" drug was exposed as dipyrone, a powerful pain-killer which can also cause a fatal blood disease called agranulocytosis. It can also cause tremors, nausea, stomach and intestinal hemorrhage and other serious side effects.

Investigation also revealed that several persons who had taken the drug had died. The harmful effects of dipyrone were well publicized in Louisiana and other states. Warnings were issued by both the American Medical Association and the Food and Drug Administration. This caused a sharp decrease in the use of dipyrone. But other powerful drugs, including cortisone derivatives, continue to be offered as cures for arthritis by clinics in Mexican border towns.

$400 MILLION WASTED EACH YEAR

According to the Arthritis Foundation, more than $400 million is spent each year by arthritis patients on worthless or harmful treatments, cures, and assorted devices. Included in the listing of worthless "nostrums" are such preparations as filtered sea water, "immune" milk, a honey and vinegar mix, alfalfa tablets, and "glorified" aspirin (a combination of aspirin and other drugs in a "secret" formula). As the Arthritis Foundation points out, "Nearly all of these are worthless, almost all are expensive, and some are actively harmful or dangerous."

Too many arthritis sufferers leap at any nostrum or device that promises relief. About 60% of all arthritis patients are tricked into buying some drug or other medication or a dietary supplement or some device with "magical powers," such as the perennial copper bracelet. Likewise they are also often lured into undergoing treatment at falsely-represented arthritis clinics.

The Arthritis Foundation offers this advice to any arthritic patient so tempted: "Be wary of any drug, device or treatment claiming to provide anything more than transient relief of minor symptoms of arthritis. Keep in mind that many medicines confining themselves to claims for temporary relief are composed primarily of aspirin or one of the salicylates. These latter drugs may be readily purchased at a fraction of the cost of the heavily advertised or glamorized product."

NO QUICK CURE, NO EASY TREATMENT

The informed arthritic patient knows that there is no quick cure or easy treatment for this disease. If you have any doubts about this or if you are tempted to try a misleadingly advertised product that promises complete relief or "cure," discuss it with your physician. You can also get reliable information from your county medical society, the local health department, or a nearby chapter of the Arthritis Foundation.

Just because a product is on the market does not mean it is worthy or reliable. When a product is misrepresented, the manufacturers and promoters are eventually involved in court proceedings. Even when legal proceedings have been initiated, they try to delay any legal action until their products have made sizeable profits.

You should also be wary of so-called "testimonials" from arthritic patients who claim to have been cured. It may be that there was a spontaneous remission of their arthritis which coincided with the taking of the touted drug or treatment, and they are giving it credit for something it has not done.

Above all, rely on the advice and treatment prescribed by your physician. Don't be duped by fraudulent claims that will delay beneficial treatment and prove a worthless and costly expense to you.

CHAPTER 13

The Promise of Research

Every arthritis sufferer should take consolation in the fact that research to discover the cause of this chronic illness has led to some promising developments. The cause has not been discovered as yet, but new theories are being formulated which may in time unlock the mysteries of this disease which has plagued scientists and physicians for centuries. And once the cause is known, finding the cure or more effective treatment will be a great deal easier than it is now.

RESEARCH IN INFLAMMATION

It is the inflammation associated with arthritis which causes the greatest amount of damage and is the greatest threat to the patient's bodily health. For these reasons a great deal of research has been done on the causes and effects of inflammation.

In the case of arthritis, a number of cells are involved in the inflammation process which, through chemical reaction, actually promote the inflammation and its damaging effects. The white blood cell is one of these. Scientists refer to the white blood cell as a "defender" cell because when there is an infection or injury somewhere in the body, for example to a joint, muscle, or surrounding tissue, the white blood cells will tend to concentrate in this area.

These white blood cells attack the foreign substances responsible for the injury or infection. In so doing, many of them are destroyed. As they are destroyed they release chemicals which can be harmful to the tissue involved. This in itself causes further inflammation.

Another type of cell, also a defender cell, becomes active in the injured or infected area. The purpose of this cell is to produce antibodies to fight the infection or to help heal the injury. But if the infection or injury is due to arthritis, for some unknown reason these defender cells produce *harmful* antibodies which actually damage the normal, as yet unaffected, substances in the joint. This also increases the inflammation.

A third cell attracted to the arthritic joint is the "scavenger" cell. The purpose of these cells, under normal conditions, is to absorb and dispose of foreign particles, disease germs, and other irritants. These scavenger cells contain colonies of powerful enzymes within tiny, sac-like bodies, called lysosomes. The material to be disposed of is passed into these enzyme-containing sacs to be digested by the enzymes.

Under normal conditions the enzymes remain within the sac or lysosome, but when arthritis is involved the enzymes escape. They then cause irritation and injury to cartilage, bones, muscles, and other tissues in the affected area. See illustration on opposite page.

The Arthritis Foundation comments, "What scientists have now discovered is that various cells, intended by nature to do good things to protect the body from trouble, actually do bad things and cause trouble in one way and another."

Current research has also shown that some of the drugs that have been used in the treatment of arthritis for many years, drugs such as aspirin, gold salts, and the corticosteroids, are useful in limiting the damaging activities of cells involved in the inflammation of arthritic joints.

CAUSED BY A VIRUS?

Researchers have recently developed a theory that arthritis is caused by a virus-like organism. This has its basis in the fact that a number of human diseases are caused by specific tiny organisms similar to viruses, which act as the infectious agent. The inflammation incident to arthritis, according to this theory, has all the characteristics of having been caused by an infection.

Advocates of this theory assert that the virus-like organism lives in the body for long periods of time without causing any problems. Then it is suddenly activated, touching off an arthritic attack. This puts the body's defense system in motion. But instead of bringing relief, as normally intended, these defender cells actually intensify the inflammation and the resultant damage to joints and tissues.

As yet, this theory has not been proved, but researchers have begun to find traces of virus-like organisms in tissue inflamed by arthri-

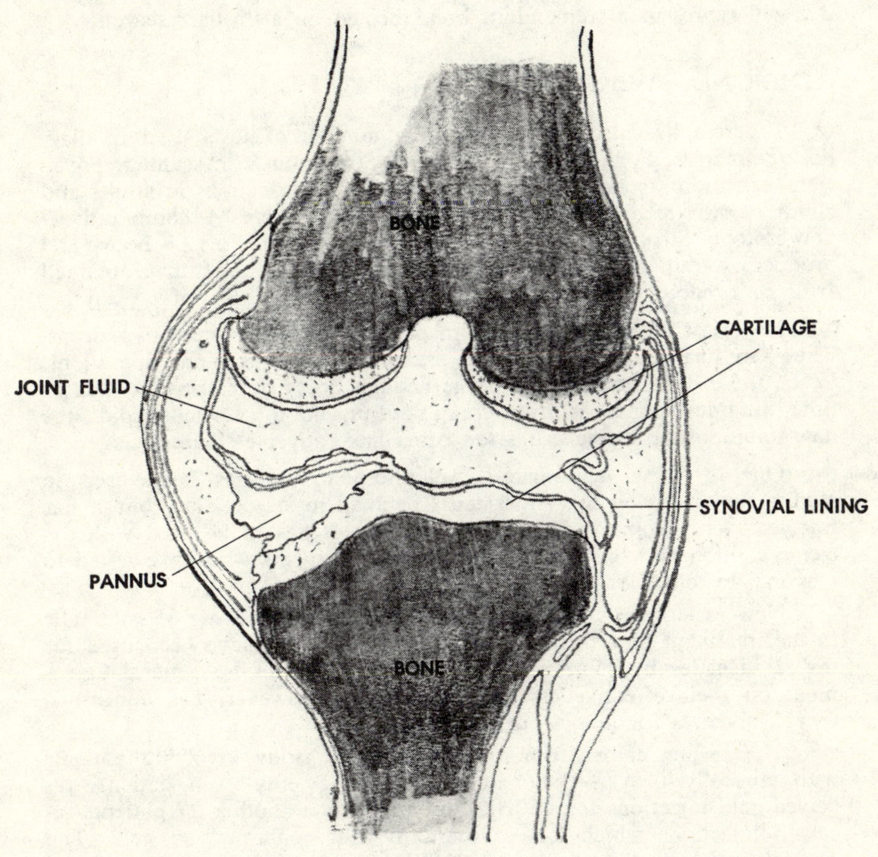

According to recent research on the causes and effects of inflammation, when a joint is inflamed the cartilage, which protects the bone ends in a joint, is eaten away and destroyed in the area of inflammation (the pannus in the drawing above). This is caused by a "rain" of enzymes from various sources and by substances released from cells which multiply and pile up on it.

tis. If the virus-like organism can be identified as the causative agent, this will represent a tremendous breakthrough in arthritis research.

OTHER NEW DEVELOPMENTS

Progress has also been made in a number of tests used in diagnosing arthritis. For example, by using a Strontium 87m scanner, physicians can more accurately detect bone and joint infections in adults and children with relative safety from radioactive effects. A comparatively new isotope, Strontium 87m has a very short half-life of 2.8 hours and produces a radiation exposure of approximately 1% of that obtained from its predecessor, Strontium 85, which has a half-life of 64 days.

Experiments are also being made with immunosuppressive drugs. These are drugs similar to those used in organ transplant operations. When these drugs are used in large enough doses over short periods of time, the improvement is often dramatic. But, like the corticosteroids, the new immunosuppressive drugs too often have adverse side effects.

One of these new drugs, cyclophosphamide, has been used in studies sponsored by the American Rheumatism Association, but it has not yet been recommended for general use. It has to be used with extreme caution and only in carefully selected patients who have failed to respond to other types of therapy.

New experiments have also been conducted in the use of gold salts in the treatment of arthritis. Even though gold salts have been used for several decades by some physicians, there has been no general agreement on their effectiveness. A recent study, however, has confirmed its effectiveness for many, but not all, patients.

The results came from a "double-blind" study involving patients with clinically proven rheumatoid arthritis. Twenty-seven patients received gold injections for up to 28 months, while another 27 patients received injections which looked the same but contained no gold. The physicians involved and their patients, all of whom volunteered for the study, did not know which patients were receiving the gold treatment and which were not (hence the designation "double blind").

In reporting the results, the Arthritis Foundation stated, "The results of this particular double-blind study were clear-cut. In a significant number of patients, gold not only relieved the symptoms of arthritis but also arrested or slowed down the disease process. These findings confirm

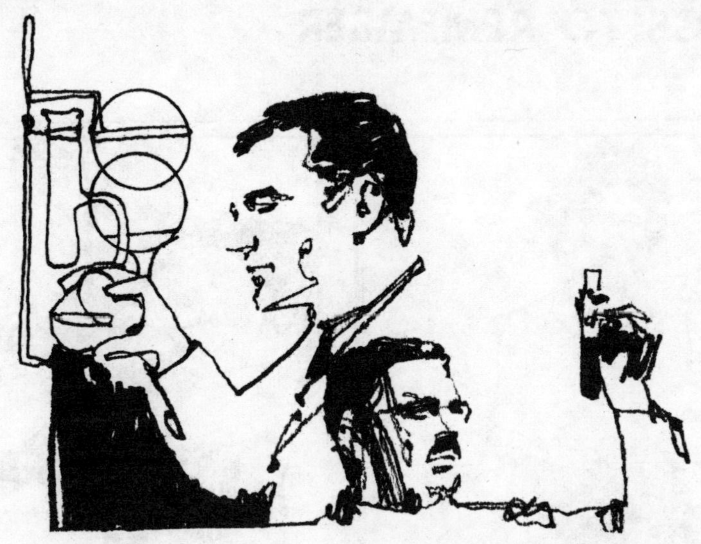

the opinion held by a large proportion of rheumatologists who have used this form of therapy for many years."

The Foundation also pointed out, however, that gold treatment may be a beneficial form of treatment for many but not for all patients with rheumatoid arthritis. Gold salts must be used with caution and under strict medical supervision because they can have a number of undesirable side effects.

REASON TO HOPE

Even as you read this, a group of researchers may be close to an important new discovery in the causes of arthritis or in the development of new drugs and methods of treatment that will bring quicker and more effective relief. Until that time, however, the only solution to the arthritis sufferer's problems is to follow his physician's advice and treatment plan faithfully and conscientiously. That is the only way your condition will improve.

You can take heart, however, in the fact that new and continuing research gives the arthritis sufferer every reason to hope that more effective drugs and methods of treatment will be forthcoming.

THINGS TO REMEMBER

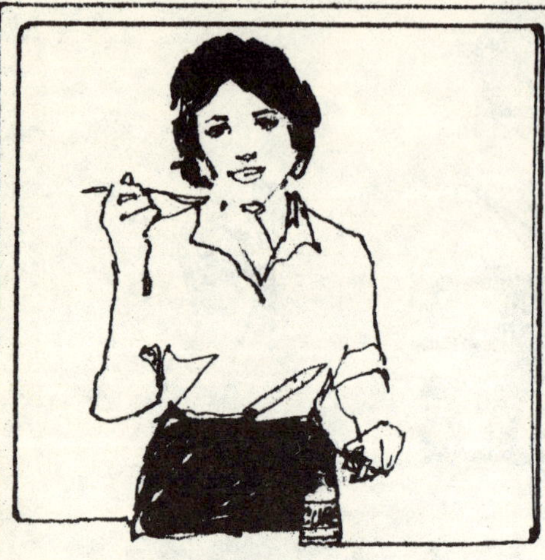

Avoid unprescribed medicines

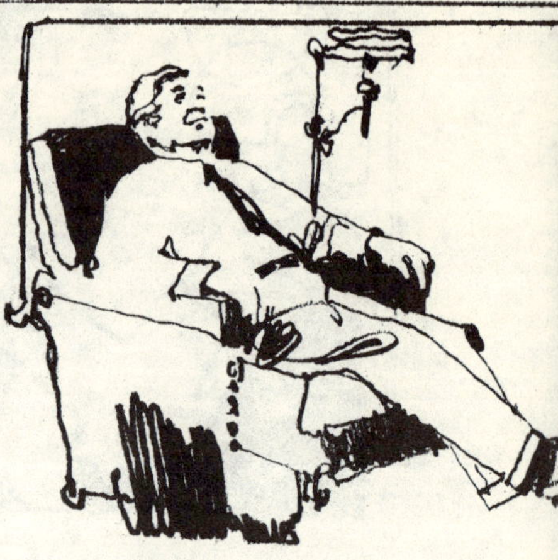

Rest and relax —physically and mentally

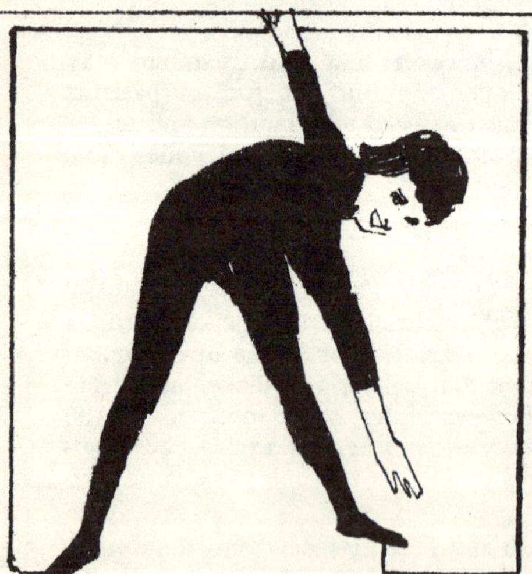

Do recommended exercises

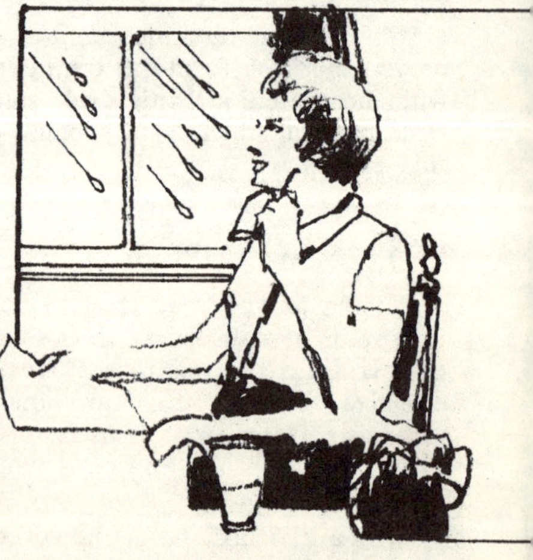

Avoid cold, wet weather

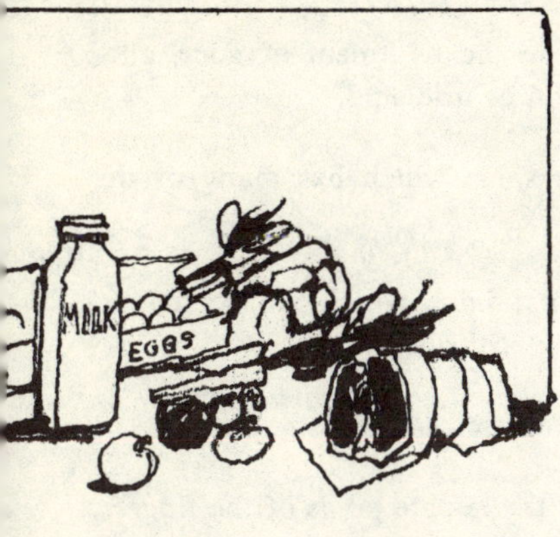

Eat a well balanced diet

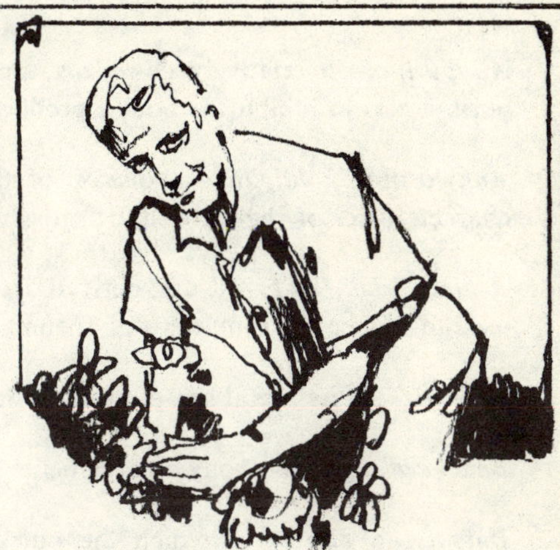

Get plenty of sunshine and heat

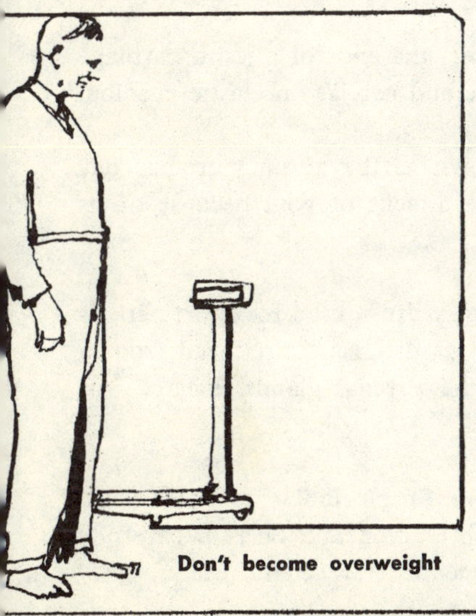

Don't become overweight

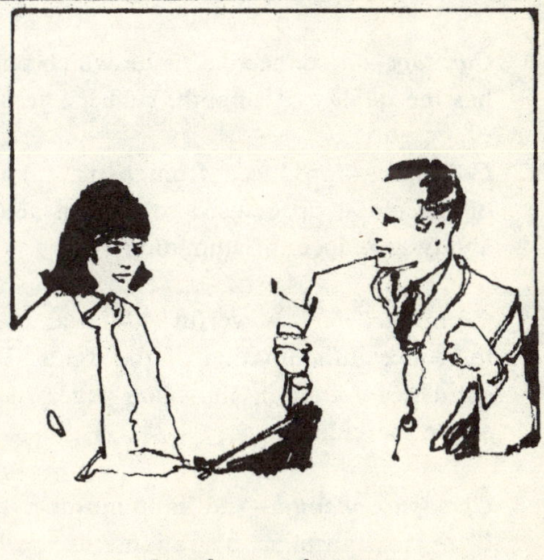

Consult your physician

Allopurinol—a relatively new drug used in the treatment of gout, allopurinol acts to inhibit the body's production of uric acid.

Ankylosing Spondylitis—a disease of the spine which has many of the characteristics of rheumatoid arthritis.

Antimalarial Drugs—drugs derived from quinine which are sometimes used to reduce the symptoms of rheumatoid arthritis.

Arthritis—in its literal sense means inflammation of a joint.

Bouchard's Nodes—bony enlargements of the middle joints of the fingers.

Bursitis—a disease in which the bursa, the small sac containing fluid which acts as a buffer between adjoining tissues within a joint structure, becomes inflamed.

Cartilage—a connective tissue which covers the ends of a joint, cartilage has the quality of smooth, rubbery gristle and acts as an elastic cushion.

Colchicine—produced from a plant known as the autumn crocus, one of the oldest drugs used to control acute attacks of gout because of its ability to reduce inflammation.

Corticosteroids—powerful anti-inflammatory drugs used for short periods to reduce inflammation of the joints. These drugs are produced from a substance found in the outer layer of the adrenal glands, located just above the kidneys.

Cyclophosphamide—an immunosupressive drug, similar to those used in organ transplant operations, used with caution and only in carefully selected arthritic patients, not yet recommended for general use.

Fibrositis—a disease involving a combination of unexplained symptoms of aches, pains, and stiffness in various parts of the body; a very difficult condition to treat.

Functional Wrist Splint—a splint designed to give support to the wrist but permitting movement of the fingers.

German Measles Syndrome—a condition in which arthritic joint pains occur in conjunction with German measles.

Gold Treatment—the use of gold salts to relieve or reduce the symptoms of arthritis.

Gout—a disease which affects the joints and kidneys, caused by abnormal body chemistries which produce an excess amount of uric acid.

Heberden's Nodes—bony enlargements of the end joints of the fingers.

Immunosuppressive Drugs—drugs similar to those used in organ transplant operations, which, like the corticosteroids, can have adverse side effects.

Indomethacin—an anti-inflammatory drug.

Liefcort—a drug banned in the United States and Canada and declared "imminently dangerous."

Ligaments—sheets and strands of dense fibers which keep the joint ends together, completely enclosing the joint in a capsule-like arrangement.

Methyl Methacrylate—a cement used to form a synthetic bone base to connect the hip or knee bones of patients with metal and plastic joints.

"Mixed" Arthritis—a term used when rheumatoid arthritis and osteoarthritis occur at the same time. This is usually caused by rheumatoid arthritis which can lead to secondary osteoarthritis due to injury to the joints.

Monosodium Urate Crystals—in gout, a uric acid salt which collects in one or more joints, causing inflammation and pain.

Osteoarthritis—a disease of the joints which involves a breakdown of cartilage and other tissues which make it possible for a joint to move normally. Inflammation may or may not be present.

Phenylbutazone—a drug used to treat acute outbreaks of arthritic pain for a short period of time.

Physiatrist—a physician who specializes in physical medicine such as developing a program of exercises for arthritic patients to help prevent crippling.

Physical Therapist or Occupational Therapist—medical personnel trained to supervise programs of exercises for arthritic patients.

Prednisone—a powerful corticosteroid sometimes used in the treatment of arthritis. It must be used under a doctor's direction to prevent serious side effects.

Primary Osteoarthritis—a term used when osteoarthritis occurs without having been influenced by any known event or injury; in other words, it started by itself.

Probenecid—a drug used to prevent the accumulation of uric acid in the body by increasing the amount of excretion of uric acid by the kidney.

Psoriatic Arthritis—a disease in which psoriasis is complicated by arthritis which has the characteristics of rheumatoid arthritis.

Purines—substances contained in foods which, through a series of chemical reactions, the body converts into uric acid.

"Referred Pain"—a term used when pain is felt some distance away from the affected joint. An example of this is an osteoarthritic hip which causes pain in the area near the patient's knees.

Reiter's Syndrome—a disease involving inflammation of the urethra, the passage through which urine is discharged from the bladder, inflammation of the delicate membrane which lines the eyelids, and arthritis in several joints.

Remission—in rheumatoid arthritis, when the disease appears to have gone away by itself. This is usually a temporary condition.

Resting Splints—splints designed to be used when the patient is resting or sleeping.

Rheumatic Fever—a disease caused by streptococcus infection which results in inflammation of the joints and may cause damage to the heart.

Rheumatism—denotes unspecific or unexplained aches and pains that may occur in joints or muscles or both. When doctors in Great Britain use the term "rheumatism" they include most forms of arthritis. In this country arthritis is more commonly used to include rheumatism as well as other similar conditions.

Rheumatoid Arthritis—inflammation of the joints in which the whole body can be affected. Symptoms include stiffness and aching of joints, general fatigue, and loss of appetite.

Rheumatologist—a physician who specializes in the treatment and management of patients with arthritis.

Secondary Osteoarthritis—a term used when osteoarthritis occurs because of wear or tear or injury to one or more joints.

Scleroderma—a disease that causes thickening and hardening of the skin, giving it a leather-like quality.

Sulfinpyrazone—one of the newer uricosuric agents used to help prevent the accumulation of uric acid in the body.

Synovial Membrane—the lining of the ligaments which secretes a slippery fluid, making it possible for joints to operate smoothly.

Systemus Lupus Erythematosus (SLE)—a disease that involves inflammation and damage to the connective tissues throughout the body.

Tophaceous Gout—a condition caused by deposits of monosodium urate monohydrate, a white, chalky compound of uric acid, which accumulate in the tissues.

Uric Acid—a chemical compound in the form of salts which is found in the joints of gout sufferers. It is also the major constituent of kidney stones.

Vitalium—an alloy composed of cobalt, chromium, and molybdenum, used in the manufacture of artificial joints.

PERSONAL NOTES

PERSONAL NOTES

PERSONAL NOTES

PERSONAL NOTES

PERSONAL NOTES

PERSONAL NOTES

PERSONAL NOTES